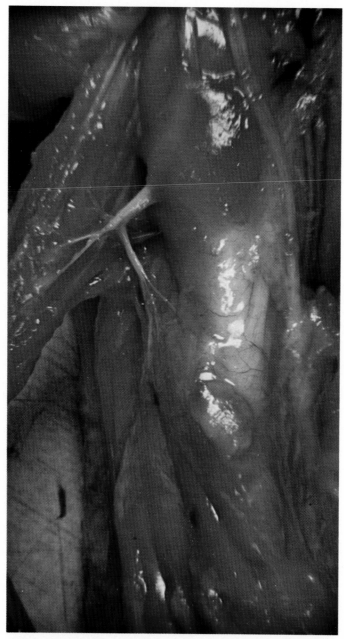

The dissection of the extensor surface of the right forearm of a full-term fetus demonstrates the passage of the posterior interosseous nerve through the supinator muscle. Note the detailed fine terminal branching of this nerve.

Morton Spinner, M.D.

Clinical Professor of Orthopaedic Surgery,
Albert Einstein College of Medicine, New York;
Chief of the Hand Surgical Service,
Department of Orthopaedic Surgery,
Brookdale Hospital Medical Center,
Brooklyn, New York

Injuries to the Major Branches of Peripheral Nerves of the Forearm

With a translation of J. Tinel's original *"Fourmillement"* Paper by Emanuel B. Kaplan, M.D.

SECOND EDITION

W. B. SAUNDERS COMPANY *Philadelphia • London • Toronto*

W. B. Saunders Company: West Washington Square
Philadelphia, PA 19105

1 St. Anne's Road
Eastbourne, East Sussex BN21 3UN, England

1 Goldthorne Avenue
Toronto, Ontario M8Z 5T9, Canada

Library of Congress Cataloging in Publication Data

Spinner, Morton.

Injuries to the major branches of peripheral nerves of
the forearm.

Includes index.

1. Forearm—Wounds and injuries.   2. Nerves, Peripheral—
Wounds and injuries.   I. Title.   II. Title: Major
branches of peripheral nerves of the forearm. [DNLM:
1. Forearm injuries.   2. Peripheral nerves—injuries.
WE820 S757i]

RD557.S65 1978   617'.1   77–16962

ISBN 0–7216–8524–2

Injuries to the Major Branches of   ISBN 0-7216-8524-2
Peripheral Nerves of the Forearm

Last digit is the print number: 9   8   7   6   5   4   3   2

*Dedicated to my loving wife, Paula
and my children,
Jeffrey
Robert
and
Steven*

PREFACE
to the Second Edition

During the 6 years following the publishing of the first edition my experience with some of the unusual problems of the forearm has increased. This text is based on 40 cases of lesions of the anterior interosseous nerve and 100 cases of lesions of the posterior interosseous nerve. They were selected from 670 peripheral nerve injuries that I have personally treated. Other unusual syndromes of neural compression lesions of the forearm, such as the pronator syndrome, are included. Localization of the lesions and differential diagnosis are stressed.

Happily, many workers in this field have contributed significantly to the literature. The bibliography has been updated to include these contributions.

A second edition is written to expand and to clarify earlier observations. Line drawings and three new sections have been added. The new sections deal with the current concept of the management of nerve compression lesions, the clinical application of electroneuromyographic procedures as applied to neural lesions of the forearm and hand, and the internervous planes of the forearm. I have added this new material in an attempt to further elucidate my presentation of the subject of injuries to major branches of peripheral nerves of the forearm. In addition, the clinical material of the older sections has been expanded.

Dr. Emanuel B. Kaplan has again been present in the background. He has given to me freely and warmly his scientific advice.

I wish to compliment Hugh Thomas for his invaluable artistic contributions to this present work.

My gratitude to Dr. Irwin R. Cohen for his untiring efforts in review of the galley and page proofs for this book.

At the Brookdale Hospital library, Ms Z. Viher and S. Winston have made new and old source material continually available to me. I am also indebted to Mr. Denis Gafney and Mrs. Ada Gams, research librarians at the New York Academy of Medicine, for their professional assistance.

Photographic technical aid has been performed by Marianné von Hooren.

I wish to thank my children, Jeffrey and Robert, for assisting me in the awesome job of typing a great portion of this manuscript.

My entire family shares in the satisfaction of having contributed to this effort through their patience and support during its preparation. I give special thanks to Paula, my wife, for having provided the love, interest and strength to help me complete this study.

Morton Spinner

PREFACE
to the First Edition

This work is limited to the various lesions of the branches of the peripheral nerves in the forearm which present problems of interpretation and treatment. While some of the lesions of these nerves were described in the past as "spontaneous non-traumatic paralysis of the posterior interosseous nerve" and "isolated anterior interosseous neuritis," the author takes a different view of their pathology and management.

During the past 15 years, I have studied these lesions both clinically and in the dissecting laboratory. I have analyzed the accumulated material and have made special studies of the anatomy of the regions in an effort to elucidate the complexities of these lesions of the forearm. This led to further attempts to place these lesions in perspective with other peripheral nerves of the forearm and their major branches.

This text represents material based on 22 cases of lesions of the anterior interosseous nerve and 45 cases of lesions of the posterior interosseous nerve responsible for paralysis. They were selected from 420 peripheral nerve injuries personally reviewed for this study. Additional injuries to other major branches of peripheral nerves in the forearm have been included.

It is hoped that this isolated study of the nerves of the forearm will help the clinician to recognize, understand, and treat some of the obscure and hard to interpret lesions of the forearm and hand.

The author is indebted to Dr. Emanuel B. Kaplan, a teacher and friend, for his role in guiding the work described in this study. His knowledge of anatomy, which spans time and language barriers, was frequently drawn upon during its preparation. I am pleased that he has permitted me to include his translation of J. Tinel's classic paper on the "tingling" sign which bears Tinel's name.

Dr. Joseph E. Milgram, as the Director of Orthopedic Surgery at the Hospital for Joint Disease, New York, encouraged the author 15 years ago to delve deeply into the problem of isolated paralysis of the long flexors of the thumb and index fingers. I wish to express my gratitude to Dr. Arthur J. Barsky for his initial suggestion that this material be presented in its entirety.

Dr. Lawrence Prutkin of New York University School of Medicine and Dr. France Baker-Cohen of the Albert Einstein College of Medicine were most helpful and cooperative in allowing me to use their anatomical laboratories for the dissections presented in this study.

My partners, Drs. Abel Kenin, Jack Levine, Bernard Freundlich, and Joel Teicher, were of assistance in bringing selected cases to my attention.

I want to convey my appreciation to Dr. Robert Weller, Donald LeVine, and Judith LeVine for their valued suggestions in editing this book. Dr. Charles Weiss was exceptionally helpful in planning the layouts for the photographic plates. Gottfried W. Goldenberg, A.M.I., prepared all the line illustrations for this text. Marianné von Hooren, MPh, converted my original color slides into black and white prints.

Mrs. Linda Katz, reference librarian, and Raymond Wright, of the interlibrary loan section of the Albert Einstein College of Medicine library staff, were most helpful in obtaining the older source material necessary for the preparation of this book.

The editors of the Journal of Bone and Joint Surgery, Clinical Orthopaedics and Related Research, and the Bulletin of the Hospital for Joint Diseases kindly permitted me to reproduce some of the text and illustrations from several of my earlier papers which have appeared in their journals.

I wish to express my gratitude to my parents, Clara and Morris Spinner, for providing me with the opportunity to study medicine.

Acknowledgments would be incomplete without a tribute to my wife, Paula, whose encouragement and understanding have helped make this study possible.

Morton Spinner

CONTENTS

Section I

HISTORICAL REVIEW

HISTORICAL REVIEW

Our knowledge concerning the physiology, anatomy, repair, and reconstruction of injured nerves has derived from work done by physicians and scientists of many nations. When one surveys the accumulated information on nerves it becomes evident that there is a joint, continuing effort being made by many investigators and clinicians. Strangely and sadly enough, wars, whether they have been between countries or within a single nation, have contributed greatly to this vast experience.

Looking back over the centuries it becomes evident that comparatively little was done on the repair of severed nerves until the last 100 years. There is evidence that Hippocrates[34] was not aware of the difference between nerves and tendons, and it has been suggested that Galen,[29] while recognizing the lesion of nerve severance, was of the opinion that a damaged nerve was irreparable.

In *Cyrurgia* (1275), a surgical text of the 13th century, an Italian surgeon, Gugliemo Salicetti, demonstrated how to repair a divided nerve, a concept which his pupil Lanfrank[17] continued to expound. In the 14th century Guy de Chauliac[6] also reapproximated severed neural tissue, and in the early years of the 17th century Ferrara (1608)[9] taught that divided nerves should be repaired. Nevertheless, the concept of nerve repair was not generally accepted until late in the 19th century.

Even though nerves had been sutured at that time, it was evident that the details of the repair process of the peripheral nerve had to be understood before an improvement in the technique could be possible. Although this work on nerve repair began with the earliest clinicians and has been carried on by a vast number of nerve physiologists, anatomists, and chemists up to the present, there is still a need for more information. Nerve function, regeneration, and chemistry still require further study and understanding.

Detailed knowledge of the peripheral nerve begins with the study of the cell body in the anterior aspect of the spinal cord. The detail concerning the structure of the cell, its dendrites, and what goes on at the cell level at the time of nerve regeneration is the end product of studies conducted by many investigators. Theodore Schwann in 1838 discovered the sheath which covers the axis cylinder of nerves and which now bears his name. Otto Deiters (1865) showed that each nerve cell has an axis cylinder and dendrites. Louis-Antoine Ranvier (1878) described the nodes of the axon cylinder, and Franz Nissl (1860–1919) described the intracellular bodies of the anterior horn cells, which are of importance in peripheral nerve regeneration.

To see all these structures, finer techniques of staining were necessary. Camillo Golgi of Italy developed the silver nitrate technique in 1873, and in 1897 the Spanish histologist Santiago Ramón y Cajal utilized his "gold salt" staining technique for nerve study. Progress in microscopic studies continues to be made with the electron microscope which magnifies structures tens of thousands of times beyond that seen by the expert histologists of the last century. Bourne,[3] Dyck,[8] Lampert, Ochoa, Spencer, Thomas, Webster — men throughout the world — are adding detailed ultrastructural information concerning the normal and pathologic states of the peripheral nervous system.

The deep interest shown by the scientific world in nerve regeneration and function and nerve impulse and physiology had its origins centuries ago. Some of the earlier pronouncements by Paré,[22] in France, indicated a pessimism concerning the possibilities of restoring nerve function. The early 19th century concept of spontaneous regeneration propounded by Wood, Velpeau, Swan, and Virchow discouraged attempts at surgical correction, which we consider so necessary today. Guthrie,[13] as late as 1827, in a *Treatise on Gunshot Wounds and Injuries* reported that he knew of no case in man in which nerve function was recovered after a main nerve was severed.

While it is hard to say who was the first person to repair a nerve in modern times, it should be noted that animal experiments concerning methods of nerve regeneration were carried out as early as 1776. In the years covering the second half of the 18th century William C. Cruikshank (1745–1800)[5] of Edinburgh, Scotland, an assistant of William Hunter, studied the return of function to a reunited severed nerve, and in 1787 J. Arnemann[1] of Germany became the first to suture a divided nerve in modern times. Unfortunately in Arnemann's study the distal segment had collapsed and regrowth did not occur.

In the early 1800's Prevost (1826)[24] demonstrated that regeneration was a very slow process, and Flourens[10] developed a technique of approximating nerves by suturing the tissue about the nerve. Augustus Volney Waller,[35] of Faversham, England, in 1850 showed that if the glossopharyngeal or hypoglossal nerves were severed, the distal segment cut off from the nerve cell underwent degeneration, while the central segment remained relatively intact. Thus the concept of "wallerian degeneration" was first proposed a little over a century ago. The studies of Ranvier, His, and Kölliker also added to the understanding of nerve regeneration.

The first of the modern suture techniques by epineural repair was performed clinically by Baudens[2] in 1836, and in 1854 Von Langenbeck[18] reported what appears to be the first successful repair of a median nerve laceration with complete return of function one year postoperatively. It was from the earliest type of clinical experimental studies carried out by Flourens and other neurohistologists of the 19th century that early surgeons gained the basic knowledge of repair and were able to apply it to clinical problems.

Neurophysiologists and neuroanatomists also have played an important role in the development of our understanding of nerves and their function and restoration. Froment, Rauber, Guyon, Frankel, Frohse, Gruber, all anatomists of the 19th century, as well as Brash,[4] Hovelacque,[16] Paturet,[23] Pitres, Testut[32] and Sunderland[31] of the 20th century, have amassed detailed gross studies of the peripheral nerves and their variations. The neurophysiologist Guillaume Duchenne (1806–1875)[7] applied faradic current in his study of muscular and nervous disorders. His *Physiology of Motion* (1862) is a landmark in clinical neurophysiology. Of the brilliant period of French clinical neurology, Charcot, Déjerine, and Marie must be mentioned for their contributions.

The difference between sensory and motor nerves was described by Bell (1826) and Magendie (1822).[11] The reflex arc studies, compounding and coordinating the whole nervous system, and the concept of reciprocal innervation between extensor and flexor muscles, were described for the first time by Charles Scott Sherrington[28] in the last decade of the 19th century. Modern neurophysiology of the peripheral nervous system has taken rapid strides through the works of Montcastle, Craine, and their confreres.

Much opportunity for research has been afforded by that bane of mankind, war. The nerve injuries of the Civil War enabled Weir Mitchell[20] to study and understand the problem of causalgia. In World War I on both sides of the line similar injuries allowed Tinel[33] of France and Hoffmann[14, 15] of Germany to add significant information concerning the recovery of injured nerves. The Tinel-Hoffmann sign of advancing unmyelinated fibrils, as they grow down the distal neural tube, was described in 1915. As a result of World War II, Seddon[27] added further knowledge on a clinical basis to the understanding of traumatic lesions of the peripheral nerve system. He also studied the results of nerve bridge grafts and cable grafts, the rate of neural regeneration and clinical evaluations of lesions at varying levels.[26] Millesi in the last 10 years has refined grafting methods. His interfunicular grafting technique offers a means of restoring neural continuity and function where recovery was impossible in the past.[19]

In recent years Moberg[21] has stressed the importance of restoration of sensation to the hand. He has demonstrated the importance of two-point discrimination and the ninhydrin tests in evaluating the return of sensory function. In the last three decades Sunderland[31] has supplied detailed information concerning the internal neuroanatomy of the peripheral nerves. Studies on this subject were started earlier in this century by the German anatomist Ranschburg[25] and the clinician Stoffel.[30]

It is impossible in this concise review to mention all of the names of important contributors to the development of neurophysiology and neuroanatomy of the peripheral nervous system. Thus, many names have been unwillingly omitted.

Basic knowledge concerning the function, structure, and repair of peripheral nerves continues to be of interest. Scientists throughout the world today are using new techniques in an attempt to bring forth additional information about the peripheral nervous system in order to restore function to damaged nerves.

BIBLIOGRAPHY

1. Arnemann, J.: Versuche über die Regeneration der Nerven. p. 221, Göttingen, Vandenhoeck et Ruprecht, 1787.
2. Baudens, J. B. L.: Clinique des Plaies d'Armes à Fèu. Paris, Ballière, 1836.
3. Bourne, G.: The Structure and Function of Nervous Tissue. New York, Academic Press, Inc., 1968.
4. Brash, J. C.: Neuro-Vascular Hila of Limb Muscles. Edinburgh, E. & S. Livingstone, 1955.
5. Cruikshank, W.: Experiments of the Nerves, Particularly on their Reproduction. Phil. Tr. Roy. Soc. Lond., 85:177–189, 1795.
6. de Chauliac, Guy: On Wounds and Fractures. Transl. by W. A. Brennan, Chicago, private printing, 1923.
7. Duchenne, G. B.: Physiology of Motion. Transl. by Emanuel B. Kaplan, M.D., Philadelphia, W. B. Saunders, 1959.
8. Dyck, P. J., Thomas, P. K., and Lambert, E. H. (eds.): Peripheral Neuropathy. 2 vols., Philadelphia, W. B. Saunders, 1975.
9. Ferrara, G.: Nuova Selva di Cirugia Divisia in Tre Parti. Venice, Combi, 1608.
10. Flourens, M. P.: Experiences sur la Réúnion ou Cicatrisation des Plaies de la Moelle Einière et des Nerfs. Ann. Sc. Nat., 13:113, 1828.
11. Garrison, F. H.: An Introduction to the History of Medicine. 4th Ed., Philadelphia, W. B. Saunders, 1929.
12. Gurdijian, E. S., and Webster, J. E.: Operative Neurosurgery. Baltimore, Williams & Wilkins, 1952.
13. Guthrie, G. J.: A Treatise on Gunshot Wounds and Nerve Injuries. 3rd Ed., London, Burgess and Hill, 1827.
14. Hoffmann, P.: Ueber eine Methode, den Erflog einer Nervennaht zu beurteilen. Med. Klinik, 11:359–360, 1915.
15. Hoffmann, P.: Weiteres über das Verhalten frisch regenerierter Nerven und über die Methode. den Erflog einer Nervennaht frühzeitig zu beurteilen. Med. Klinik, 11:856–858, 1915.
16. Hovelacque, A.: Anatomie des Nerfs Craniens et Rachidiens et du Système Grand Sympathique. Paris, Doin, 1927.
17. Lanfrank: Science of Cirurgie. Early English Text Society, original series 102, p. 360, New York, Scribner, 1894.
18. Langenbeck, B. von: Verhandl. d. deutsch. Gesselsch. f. Chir. (Fünfter Congress), pp. 111–112, 1876.
19. Millesi, H., Meissl, G., and Berger, A.: Further Experience with Interfascicular Grafting of the Median, Ulnar, and Radial Nerves. J. Bone Joint Surg., 58A:209–218, 1976.
20. Mitchell, S. W.: Injuries of Nerves and their Consequences. Philadelphia, Lippincott, 1872.
21. Moberg, E.: Objective Methods for Determining the Functional Value of Sensibility in the Hand. J. Bone Joint Surg., 40B:454–476, 1958.
22. Paré, A.: The Workes of that Famous Chirurgion Ambroise Parey. Transl. by T. Johnson, London, Cotes and Dugard, 1649.
23. Paturet, G.: Traité d'Anatomie Humaine. Paris, Masson, 1951.
24. Prevost, cited by Holmes, W.: The Repair of Nerves by Suture. J. Hist. Med., 6:44, 1951.
25. Ranschburg, P.: Über die Anastomosen der Nerven der oberen Extremität des Menschen mit Rücksicht auf ihre Neurologische und Nerven Chirurgische. Bedentung. Neurol. Centralbl., 36:521–534, 1917.
26. Seddon, H. J., Medawar, P. B., and Smith, H.: Rate of Regeneration of Peripheral Nerves in Man. J. Physiol., 102:191–215, 1943.
27. Seddon, H. J.: Peripheral Nerve Injuries. Medical Research Council Report Series Number 282, London, H.M.S.O., 1954.
28. Sherrington, C. S.: The Integrative Action of the Nervous System. New York, Scribner, 1906.
29. Souques, A.: Étapes de la Neurologie dans L'Antiquité Grécque. (D'Homère A. Galien). Paris, Masson, 1936.
30. Stoffel, A.: Beitrage zur einer Rationellen Nervenchirurgie, München. Med. Wochenschr., 60:175–179, 1913.
31. Sunderland, S.: Nerves and Nerve Injuries. Baltimore, Williams & Wilkins, 1968.
32. Testut, J.: Traité d'Anatomie Humaine. 9th Ed., Paris, Doins, 1949.
33. Tinel, J.: Nerve Wounds. Symptomatology of Peripheral Nerve Lesions Caused by War Wounds. Transl. by F. Rothwell and revised by C. A. Joll, New York, Wood, 1918.
34. Walker, E. A.: History of Neurological Surgery. Baltimore, Williams & Wilkins, 1951.
35. Walker, A.: Experiments on the Section of the Glossopharyngeal and Hypoglossal Nerves of the Frog, and Observations of the Alteration Produced Thereby in the Structure of Their Primitive Fibres. Phil. Tr. Roy. Soc. Lond., 140:423–429, 1850.

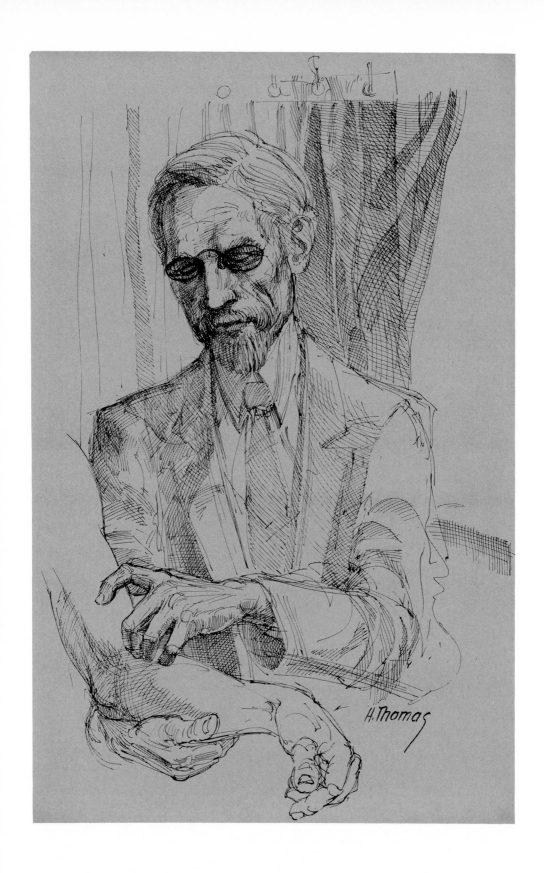

H. Thomas

Section II

J. TINEL'S "FOURMILLEMENT" PAPER

J. TINEL'S "FOURMILLEMENT" PAPER*

As a follow-up to the historical introduction, it seems appropriate and useful to present the complete translation of Tinel's study on the well-known "tingling" sign observed in nerve regeneration.

The "Tingling" Sign in Peripheral Nerve Lesions

by J. Tinel

Translated by Dr. Emanuel B. Kaplan

It is recognized that it is frequently difficult to make a precise diagnosis in lesions of peripheral nerves.

Is there a division of the nerve, a compression, a tear, or an irritation? Is the nerve in a state of regeneration? Is a palpable neuroma penetrated by axons? Was a nerve suture successful? These are the problems which confront the clinician and are of major importance in diagnosis and treatment.

Pressure applied to an injured nerve trunk frequently produces a sensation of tingling transmitted to the periphery of the nerve and localized to a precise cutaneous region.

We consider that the systematic study of the tingling produced by pressure on a nerve may bring precious help for the solution of the problems.

It is important to differentiate this frequently present tingling from a sensation of pain which may also be produced by pressure applied to the injured nerve. *Pain* is a sign of *irritation of the nerve; tingling* is a sign of *regeneration,* or more precisely, tingling reveals the presence of regenerating axons.

The *pain of nerve irritation* is almost always present as a localized pain felt at the point where pressure is applied. If it extends along the nerve trunk, it is most intense at the point of pressure. It is associated almost constantly with pain produced by pressure of the muscles, and most frequently the muscular pain is more pronounced than the pain along the nerve trunk.

---

*Tinel, J.: Le Signe du "Fourmillement" dans les Lésions des Nerfs Périphériques. Press. Med., 47:388–389, Oct. 1915.

The *tingling of regeneration* is not a painful sensation. It is a vaguely disagreeable feeling; the patient compares it with a sensation of electrical shock. This is hardly felt at the point of compression but is felt most frequently in the corresponding skin distribution. The muscles adjacent to the nerve where tingling is found are not painful.

The two types of sensation produced by pressure of the nerve — pain and tingling — are easily differentiated in almost all cases. The two sensations rarely exist simultaneously in the same nerve or, more exactly, at the same point of an examined nerve because, as we will see later, they may follow one another along the same nerve trunk. The two different signs produced by pressure applied to the nerve are similar to the symptoms which are revealed by examination of skin sensation. Regeneration of the nerve is manifested by paresthesias of a more constant type which are more painful and are associated with hypoesthesia produced by touch, by puncture and, especially, by slight friction of the skin.

However, in all cases the symptoms produced by pressure of the nerve — pain which indicates the irritation of the axons or tingling which indicates their regeneration — are much easier to differentiate than the signs of cutaneous sensibility. They are also more constant and appear much earlier; they furnish more precise, more localized and more important information.

A systematic study of tingling produced by pressure applied to the nerve frequently permits the clinician:

To establish whether there is complete or incomplete interruption of the nerve;

To determine the exact site and extent of the lesion;

To reveal early regeneration of the axons and to follow their progress and disclose their importance.

A few illustrations are presented:

1. In total nerve interruption along the course of the nerve trunk a definite zone can be found where pressure produces tingling in the cutaneous distribution of the nerve.

This zone of tingling is not extended. It does not exceed 2–3 centimeters; it is constant and absolutely fixed; it persists for weeks and months; it is confined to the course of the nerve only, and there is no extension either proximal or distal to the lesion where pressure could produce tingling.

This zone indicates that at this precise point the suddenly interrupted axons have undergone local regeneration and, being unable to cross the obstacle or find the distal segment, they wound up into a more or less large neuroma.

2. In complete interruptions of the nerve produced by very tight entrapment, the same characteristics of fixation, of permanence and precise limitation are found, but the zone of tingling is more extended; it

may reach 6, 8 or 10 centimeters more over the course of the nerve. For instance, in frequent compressions of the radial nerve associated with fractures of the humerus, it is possible by studying the tingling along the entire length of the nerve to determine if the nerve is caught in the bone callus or is interrupted at the level of the superior or inferior level of the fracture.

It is necessary to mention that simple pressure of a nerve caught in a bone callus does not produce tingling easily. The tingling is better revealed by percussion applied to the callus.

In any case, if the zone of tingling remains fixed and does not pass the inferior limits of the callus, or, if after many weeks tingling does not spread distal to the callus, it means that the entrapment produced a sufficient stricture of the nerve to interrupt the regeneration of the axons and prevents them from passing through.

3. It is possible in certain instances to find along the course of the same nerve two different sites of tingling corresponding to two different lesion levels.

For instance, we have seen two wounded men with radial nerve paralysis in the upper part of the arm. There was one zone of tingling of the radial nerve at the level of the bullet exit over the posterior aspect of the arm; there was another zone of tingling, more extended, over the lateral side of the arm at the level of a very large fracture callus; these two zones were fixed and limited. No tingling could be produced distal to the fracture site. Surgical intervention showed that the nerve was partially destroyed by the passage of the bullet and that a few fibers which escaped injury were found more distal and were compressed and interrupted in the fracture callus.

It is also possible to observe partial tingling of the nerve. Pressure of the sciatic nerve, for instance, may show a lesion limited to the medial or lateral side which will accordingly produce a tingling sensation localized in the cutaneous distribution of the common popliteal or the posterior tibial nerve.

Another instance presented a man with paralysis due to a wound over the middle of the thigh which presented a double area of tingling. Pressure applied to the nerve at the wound level produced tingling over the sole of the foot which corresponded to the posterior tibial, but pressure applied distal to the wound produced tingling in an area which reached the popliteal space and extended over the dorsum of the foot in the zone of the lateral peroneal nerve. In this case, a complete interruption of the posterior tibial component of the sciatic nerve with nonadvancing tingling was found. In addition, an incomplete interruption of the lateral part of the nerve was present with a progressive transmission of tingling through the regenerated axons down toward the popliteal space.

4. In effect, incomplete interruption of a nerve or, more exactly, lesions permitting the passage of regenerating axons are characterized by progressive extension of the tingling.

Accordingly, tingling can be seen to appear distal to the lesion, extending progressively toward the periphery along the course of the nerve. A nerve which demonstrates tingling below the lesion is a partially or totally regenerating nerve. It is possible to see the progress from week to week and thus follow the slow progress of regeneration of the axons. One may assess the speed of regeneration of the nerve and possibly judge its importance according to the intensity of tingling and the extent of the area of cutaneous response.

This also pertains to nerve sutures where it is possible by observing the progressive extension of tingling to quickly determine the success of the intervention.

Gradually, as the tingling extends and increases in intensity toward the periphery it tends to decrease and even to disappear at the site of the original injury. Thus, tingling extends eccentrically, always preserving a wide area.

Therefore, it is always necessary to explore the nerve along its entire course. The following case illustrates this principle. We examined a man who had a complete paralysis of the sciatic nerve. Five months previously he had been wounded at the proximal end of the thigh. A complete paralysis had developed since then, but the muscle tone was not completely gone and the zone of anesthesia appeared somewhat reduced. Tingling could not be found over the sciatic nerve at the level of the injury or distal to it. We thought that this indicated a poor prognosis. But on further examination we found some tingling over the popliteal space and the upper half of the leg corresponding to the branches distal to the level of injury of the nerve. This indicated that the nerve was in a stage of advanced regeneration. In effect, we could find some contractility under faradic stimulation over some fibers of the gastrocnemii, peronei and tibialis anterior.

5. The same progressive extension of the tingling zone is found in incomplete interruption with nerve irritability.

It appears that sometimes, however rarely, the signs of irritation and of regeneration are found in the same nerve; the interpretation is then quite difficult. However, generally speaking, the patient complains of a radiating painful numbness or painful pricking rather than a tingling.

In the majority of cases, however, tingling progressively replaces the pain produced by compressing the nerve. Tingling, figuratively speaking, pushes the pain away. In accordance with the advancement of tingling, the nerve trunk and the muscles become less painful. It is found that a sciatic nerve, which becomes painless, tingles on pressure of the thigh, while the nerve and the muscular masses of the leg are still painful.

It is easy to see, as illustrated by the few examples, how helpful the sign of tingling can be.

It is obvious that the systematic search of this sign does not eliminate in any way a careful examination of motor disturbances and the electrical sensory, and trophic changes. This sign is simply used in addition to the other observations and, in the majority of cases, only confirms the diagnosis and makes more precise the clinical findings.

It would indeed be unwise to overestimate the importance of the tingling sign, especially when the sign is absent. Thus it is important to mention the following points:

1. Tingling induced by pressure of the nerve does not appear generally before the 4th and even the 6th week after trauma.

In effect it is known that each nerve lesion, section or entrapment is followed by the first phase of degeneration—descending wallerian degeneration —which extends to the end of the nerve, and ascending degeneration or retrograde which does not extend beyond several nerve segments. Even when limited they are accompanied by deep changes in the cells which give origin to the nerve. It is only after this first phase of degeneration that fibrillation of the axons of the central end, and their regrowth begins. It appears that in man this phase of regeneration does not appear earlier than after 3 or 4 weeks; it appears earlier or later according to the age, the state of health and the regenerative factors of each individual. It is this period of new axon formation which corresponds to the first appearance of tingling.

2. Equally the tingling disappears as soon as the nerve returns to its normal structure and the newly formed axons become mature. Generally, it is at the end of 8 or 10 months that tingling appears to stop; wide variations are naturally observed according to individuals, lesions and the length of degenerating nerve. We have already mentioned that tingling disappears in an eccentric manner running progressively toward the periphery (distal end) of the nerve.

3. Finally, tingling may be absent in certain rare cases. Then, it indicates either that the lesion is very mild and that it did not produce any deep destruction of the nerve fibers or, on the contrary, that no regeneration occurred, as is observed at times in older individuals and patients with long illnesses or with disturbing nutritional problems.

Tingling therefore, does not constitute an absolutely constant fixed sign which is easy to interpret. It cannot replace precise and repeated examinations of the patient. It is valuable only in association with the total sum of other clinical symptoms.

With all these reservations, nevertheless, tingling appears to help clarify at times certain diagnostic neurological problems and to furnish precise indications for prognosis and treatment of peripheral nerve lesions.

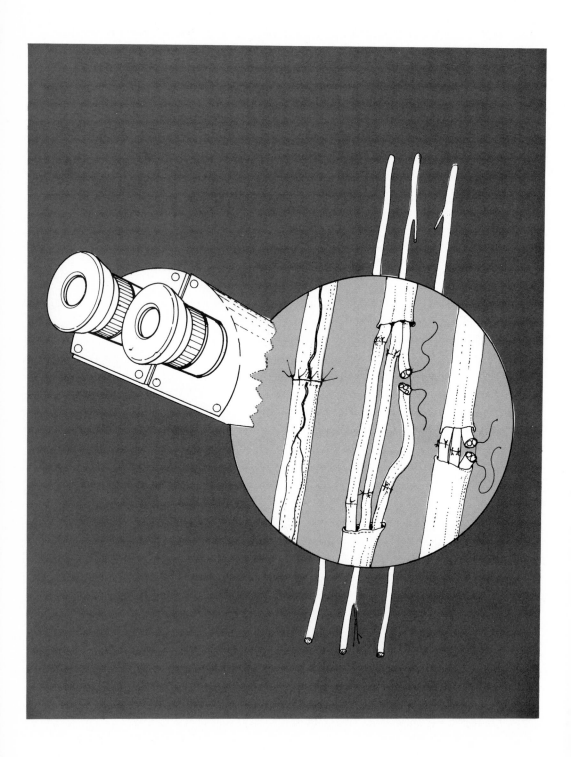

DEVELOPMENT OF MODERN TECHNIQUE OF NERVE REPAIR

DEVELOPMENT OF MODERN TECHNIQUE OF NERVE REPAIR

Our present concept of end-to-end funicular repair of a divided nerve using fine suture material and ocular magnification (Fig. 1) has been developed gradually and not without exhaustive trial and error. The modern technique has a distinct, traceable evolution.

Historically, the first modern neural repair by Baudens (1836)[4] followed the earlier experimental studies of Flourens,[12] in which the nerve sutures were passed through the epineurium. In 1870 Philipeaux and Vulpian[29] proposed a central suture technique, and in 1882 Mikulicz[27] resorted to an end-to-end repair using a "sling" suture.

While these techniques were being tried, other experiments were being carried on. Létiévant (1873)[23] proposed that local nerve flaps be used to bridge a neural defect, while in 1885 Rawa[30] tried unsuccessfully to repair a severed nerve by side-to-side coaptation. In other experiments, nerves were cut obliquely and repaired. Neuromatous bulbs were sutured end to end, or a wedge was cut in the bulb and the opposite end sewn into the slit. At one time, when a gap in the nerve existed, mere alignment of the separated ends with a suture was recommended. The regenerating nerve ends were thought to grow along the suture into the distal segment. All these techniques failed.

As new techniques for nerve repair were tried, the type of suture material changed during the years, from split tortoise tendon to 10–0 virgin silk with swaged cutting needles. Linen, hair, kangaroo tendon, catgut, silver wire, tantalum, autogenous plasma,[42] chemical splicing (methyl-2-cyanoacrylate and ethyl-2-cyanoacrylate), tubular splicing (artery, vein, millipore, silicone, gelatin on collagen film),[6, 8, 10, 26] cotton, and dacron have all been used at different times. Most have been discarded for various reasons. The most frequent cause for this is failure to achieve axon regeneration, due to severe foreign body and inflammatory response to the suture material. Currently, synthetic absorbable polyglycolic acid sutures are being evaluated. They have proved successful in restoring neural continuity in an experimental model.[18, 19]

We take for granted today the various modern methods of sterilizing suture material. From the present perspective some of the procedures used in the past seem highly unusual. For example, at one time, hot red wine served as a sterilizing fluid through which tortoise tendon was

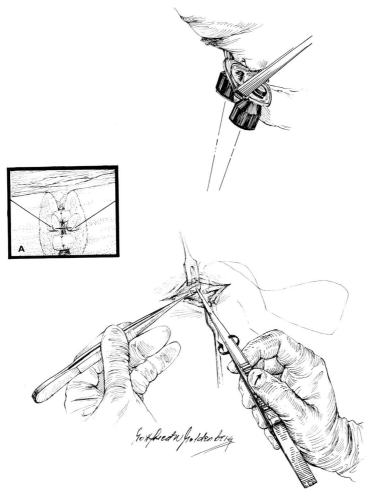

Figure 1.   The present concept of nerve repair: fine suture material, ocular magnification and funicular repair technique (A).

passed before it was used. Carbolized catgut was also used as a suture material but its use was short lived.

As experimentation in nerve repair continued, it became evident that the accurate approximation of the ends of the nerve was of paramount importance. Methods for managing nerve gaps developed slowly, with much attention directed to the amount of traction applied to the nerve ends. Maximal traction on the nerve was shown to result in intraneural hemorrhage and fibrosis, with subsequent failure of the repair, and the two-stage nerve bulb traction technique, recommended in World War II, did not pass the test of time.

As early as 1888 Schüller[33] had recommended a combination of gentle nerve stretching with optimal positioning of the joint as a means of bridging a nerve gap. Stookey (1922),[39] while pointing out that the natural slack of a nerve could be utilized to close the gap, cautioned against overstretching the nerve. In recent years, James Smith[35, 36] has proposed that gentle longitudinal traction on the neural bulb (covered with gauze) be applied in order to restore the normal length of the retracted nerve. Thus restoration of the proximal nerve segment to its pre-injury length has been viewed as an important concept in nerve repair. Aside from stressing the nerve length, Smith described the details of the vascular mesentery and emphasized that the nerve ends should not be deprived of their circulation by clearing away more than 2.5 cm. of the mesentery, otherwise a devitalized tube graft would result.

Other methods of bridging a nerve gap have been suggested and tried, such as shortening a bone (thereby shortening a limb) in order to make up for major neural tissue loss. However, this technique, whose major proponents were Löbker (1891)[24] and Dandy (1943),[9] has had limited use.

Transferring or transposing a nerve segment as a means of managing a nerve gap has received a great deal of attention through the years. The first nerve graft, though technically a failure, is accredited to Albert (1885).[1] The first successful nerve graft (for a gap in the median nerve) is said to have been performed by Robson (1889).[31] Transposition of the ulnar nerve anterior to the elbow was recommended by Gardner (1891),[14] and similar transpositions for the radial and median nerve were recommended by Wrede (1916).[46] Bunnell,[7] Ballance and Duel,[3] Seddon,[34] and Millesi[28] must also be noted for their work in nerve grafting. In recent years irradiated nerve grafts have been utilized but the current technique has produced equivocal results. Taylor and Ham[43] have described a free microsurgical nerve graft technique in which the superficial radial nerve graft is sutured and the accompanying radial artery and venae comitantes are anastomosed.

In some instances, the loop technique between irreparably damaged median and ulnar nerves, as described by Strange[40, 41] to gap a major segmental loss of the median nerve, has proved useful. Edgerton[11] adopted this concept for a patient in whom both upper extremities were involved; he used a cross arm nerve pedicle to restore vital median nerve sensory function to one hand, using the damaged proximal ulnar segment of the opposite arm.

In the last decade, because of continued interest in improving the results of nerve repair, significant changes in techniques have been proposed. The funicular reapproximation methods of Goto,[15] Bora,[5] Ito,[20] Hakstian,[17] Tsuge,[44] Freilinger,[13] and Grabb[11] have gained in popularity. Grabb has shown that one need not stimulate the funiculi proximally and distally to align motor and sensory fibers, but rather need just realign the bundles by their size and location in order to reestablish the internal topography. Freilinger et al. have developed a histochemical technique to help differentiate sensory and motor funiculi.[13] Motor fibers have a higher amount of acetylcholinesterase. The technique identifies the funicular location of this enzyme. In its current state, this intraoperative technique has limited use, as it requires two operative procedures.

It is important to note that there is frequent interchange of fibers from one funiculus to another throughout the nerve. Primary repair in which little nerve tissue must be excised offers the best opportunity to restore the funicular pattern accurately. When more than 5 mm. of the peripheral nerve on both sides is excised it may be impossible to re-establish perfectly the normal funicular pattern. In secondary neurorrhaphy, the older type of epineural repair may be the only feasible method of coaptating the nerve ends (Fig. 2). Ancillary intraoperative electrical techniques have been developed that help to evaluate a neural lesion-in-continuity of a whole nerve[21, 22] and funicular level.[45] By recording across the lesion, axons of sufficient maturity to conduct nerve action potentials distal to the site of injury can be determined well before electromyographic evidence of recovery can be demonstrated. The extent of the axon population recovery can be correlated percentagewise with the nerve action potential amplitude of the distal segment as compared with the proximal. Single fascicular electrical recordings offer the most critical intraoperative evaluation of partial neural lesions. With these intraoperative confirmatory aids, the extent of questionable lesions-

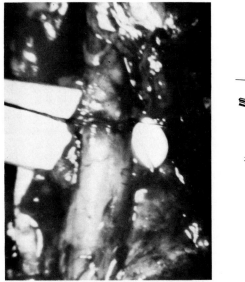
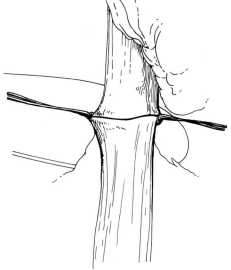

Figure 2.   A median nerve at the wrist is repaired with an epineural suture technique. Key corner stitches have been placed.

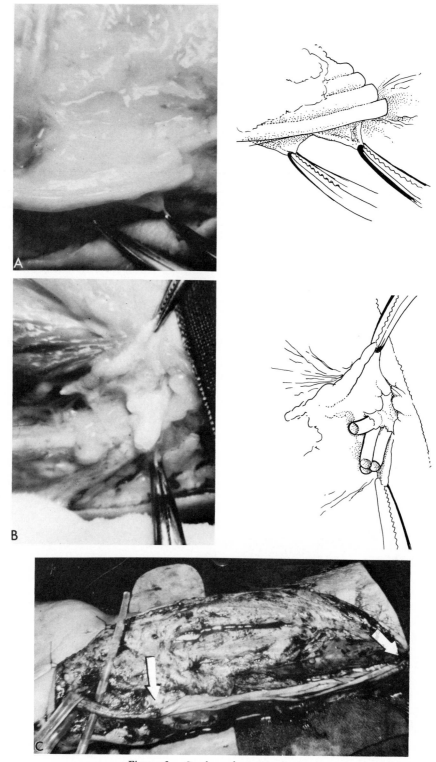

Figure 3.   *See legend on opposite page.*

in-continuity can be further assessed and the need for neural repair or neurolysis determined.

Where the funiculi can be identified and matched they are sutured with fine 8–0 to 10–0 nylon on small swaged cutting needles. The dissecting microscope or ocular loupes are used when branches of major nerves are injured near their bifurcation from the major peripheral nerve. The funicular representation of the branch can usually be teased out from the main nerve trunk and repaired accurately. The branch usually follows a 2.5-cm. intraneural course near its termination before proximal interfunicular interchange begins.

This concept of opening the epineural sheath of a damaged nerve to re-establish nerve continuity is vital in partial injuries of peripheral nerves, especially at the termination of the major peripheral nerve. Injuries of the median nerve just distal to the carpal tunnel, of the ulnar nerve in Guyon's tunnel, or of the radial nerve at the distal region of the supinator can best be managed by opening the proximal nerve trunk in order to identify and match the severed funiculi. This is most accurately and technically accomplished when these nerves are repaired primarily.

Millesi recommends that the epineurium be excised because of its scar-forming potential, and that interfunicular grafts be utilized to remove tension from the nerve suture line (Fig. 3). His results are most encouraging in cases in which the nerve gap cannot be overcome by physiological joint positioning without tension. There is excellent evidence that the thin free interfunicular grafts revascularize and act as good neural conduits.[2]

Much basic information about peripheral nerves has been accumulated during the last century. A large number of myths and misbeliefs have not passed the test of time. No longer do we believe that convulsions are caused by wounded nerves in continuity. No longer do we use ointments made of ground earthworms in the treatment of severed nerves. No longer do we use red hot irons to consolidate the ends of nerves.

Figure 3. *A* and *B*, Proximal and distal stumps of the ulnar nerve in the forearm have been prepared for interfascicular grafting. Four bundles have been step-cut at different levels. The epineurium in the hemostats will be excised. *C*, A 14 cm. defect in the ulnar nerve has been bridged utilizing the Millesi interfascicular graft technique. Proximal and distal suture sites are indicated (arrows). The donor nerve utilized was the sural nerve. (From Omer, G., and Spinner, M.: Peripheral nerve testing and suture techniques. *In* American Academy of Orthopaedic Surgeons Instructional Course Lectures, St. Louis, C. V. Mosby, 1975, Vol. 24.)

Present knowledge points to the following as the best available standards for obtaining optimum results: accuracy of funicular alignment, repair with the finest atraumatic suture, use of minimal tension, and production of minimal scarring.

Nevertheless, critical analysis of the results of nerve suture indicates that further improvement is necessary, especially in the management of the nerve wound in the adult patient. Our most dramatic successes in neural repair are concentrated in the group of patients under 20 years of age.

As vital as it is to have the best technique for nerve repair, it is equally important to know if the neural cell is dead. This knowledge is very important in proximal nerve lesions, and especially with electrical damage. As yet there is no way that the clinician can evaluate the status of the cellular pump, which is so essential for the regeneration of the axon. It certainly would help the treating physician to know early after peripheral nerve injury if the neural cell body will be capable of producing the essential substances needed. Function can be restored early by tendon transfers or by sensory substitutions if the lack of vitality of the cell is known. Non-invasive tests and techniques are needed to supply this information. Unfortunately, these are not available today.

BIBLIOGRAPHY

1. Albert, E.: Einige Operationen an Nerven. Wien. Med. Presse, 26:1221–1224, 1285–1288, 1885.
2. Almgren, K. G.: Revascularization of Free Peripheral Nerve Grafts. An Experimental Study in Rabbits. Acta Orthop. Scand. Suppl. 154, 1974.
3. Ballance, C.A., and Duel, A.B.: The Operative Treatment of Facial Palsy. Arch. Otolaryng., 15:1–70, 1932.
4. Baudens, J.B.L.: Clinique des Plaies d'Armes à Fèu. Paris, Ballière, 1836.
5. Bora, Jr., F.W.: Peripheral Nerve Repair in Cats: The Fascicular Stitch. J. Bone Joint Surg., 49A:659–666, 1967.
6. Braun, R.M.: Comparative Studies of Neurorrhaphy and Sutureless Peripheral Nerve Repair. Surg. Gynecol. Obstet., 122:15–18, 1966.
7. Bunnell, S.: Surgical Repair of the Facial Nerve. Arch. Otolaryngol., 25:235–239, 1937.
8. Campbell, J.B., Bassett, C.A.L., Husby, J., Thulin, C-A., and Feringa, E.A.: Microfilter Sheaths in Peripheral Nerve Surgery. A Laboratory Report and Preliminary Clinical Study. J. Trauma, 1:139–157, 1961.
9. Dandy, W.E.: A Method of Restoring Nerves Requiring Resection. J.A.M.A., 122:35–36, 1943.
10. Ducker, T.B., and Hayes, G.J.: Experimental Improvements in the use of Silastic Cuff for Peripheral Nerve Repair. J. Neurosurg., 28:582–587, 1967.
11. Edgerton, M.T.: Cross-Arm Nerve Pedicle Flap for Reconstruction of Major Defects of the Median Nerve. Surgery, 64:248–263, 1968.
12. Flourens, M.P.: Experiences sur la Réunion ou Cicatrisation des Plaies de la Moelle Einière et des Nerfs. Ann. Sc. Nat., 13:113, 1828.
13. Freilinger, G., Gruber, H., Holle, J., and Mandl, H.: Zur Methodik Sensomotorisch differenzierter Faszikelnaht peripherer Nerven. Handchirurgie, 7:133–137, 1975.
14. Gardner, W.: Gunshot Wound of the Arm; Resection of the Ulnar Nerve; Suture after Displacement; Recovery. Lancet, 2:808–809, 1891.
15. Goto, Y.: Experimental Study of Nerve Autografting by Funicular Suture. Arch. Jap. Chir., 36:478–494, 1967.

16. Grabb, W.C.: Management of Nerve Injuries in the Forearm and Hand. Orthop. Clin. N. Amer., *1:*2, 419–431, 1970.
17. Hakstian, R.W.: Funicular Orientation by Direct Stimulation. J. Bone Joint Surg., *50A:*1178–1186, 1968.
18. Hudson, A.R., Bilbao, J.M., and Hunter, D.: Polyglycolic Acid Suture in Peripheral Nerve: An Electron Microscopic Study. Canad. J. Neurol. Sci., *2:*17–21, 1975.
19. Hudson, A.R., and Hunter, D.: Polyglycolic Acid Suture in Peripheral Nerve. II. Sutured Sciatic Nerve. Canad. J. Neurol. Sci., *3:*69–72, 1976.
20. Ito, T.: Cited by Grabb, W.C.: Management of Nerve Injuries in the Forearm and Hand. Orthop. Clin. N. Amer., *1:*2, 419–431, 1970.
21. Kline, D.G., Hackett, E.R., and May, P.R.: Evaluation of Nerve Injuries by Evoked Potentials and Electromyography. J. Neurosurg., *31:*128–136, 1969.
22. Kline, D.G., and Nulsen, F.E.: The Neuroma in Continuity. Surg. Clin. North Am., *52:*1189–1209, 1972.
23. Létiérant, E.: Traité des Sections Nerveuses. Paris, Baillière, 1873.
24. Löbker, K.: Über die Kontinuitätsresektion de Knocken Behufs Ausführung Sekundärer Séhnen-und Nervennaht, Zentralbl. f. Chir., *11:*841–845, 1884.
25. Marmor, L.: Regeneration of Peripheral Nerves by Irradiated Homografts. J. Bone Joint Surg., *46A:*338–394, 1964.
27. Mikulicz: Cited by Schramm, H.: Beitrage zur Kaswistik und Technik der Nervennaht. Wien. Med. Wochenschr., *33:*1161–1164, 1194–1196, 1883.
28. Millesi, H.: The Interfascicular Nerve-Grafting of the Median and Ulnar Nerves. J. Bone Joint Surg., *54A:*727–750, 1972.
29. Philipeaux, J.M., and Vulpian, A.: Note sur des Essais de greffe d'un Troncon du Nerf Lingual entre les deux Bouts du Nerf Hypoglosse, après Excision d'un Segment de ce Dernier Neft. Arch. Physiol. Norm. et Path., *3:*618–620, 1870.
30. Rawa, A.L.: Ueber die Nervennaht. Wien. Med. Wochenschr., *35:*358–359, 1885.
31. Robson M.: Nerve-grafting. Brit. M.J., *2:*1312–1314, 1889.
32. Schnitker, M.T.: A Technique for Transplant of the Musculospiral Nerve in Open Reduction of Fractures of the Mid-Shaft of the Humerus. J. Neurosurg., *6:*113–117, 1949.
33. Schüller, A.: Die Verwendung der Nervendehnung zur Operativen Heilung von Substranzverlusten am Nerven. Wien. Med. Presse. No. 5 Jahrg., *29:*146–151, 1888.
34. Seddon, H.J.: The Use of Autogenous Grafts for the Repair of Large Gaps in Peripheral Nerves. Brit. J. Surg., *35:*151–167, 1947.
35. Smith, J.W.: Factors Influencing Nerve Repair. I. Blood Supply to Peripheral Nerves. Arch. Surg., *93:*335–341, 1966.
36. Smith, J.W.: Factors Influencing Nerve Repair. II. Collateral Circulation of the Peripheral Nerves. Arch. Surg., *93:*433–437, 1966.
37. Snyder, C.C., Browne, E.Z., Herzog, B.G., Johnson, E.A., and Coleman, D.A.: Epineural Cuff Neurorrhaphy. J. Bone Joint Surg., *56A:*1092, 1974.
38. Spurling, R.G.: The Use of Tantalum Wire and Foil in the Repair of Peripheral Nerves. Surg. Clin. N. Amer., *23:*1491–1504, 1943.
39. Stookey, B.: Surgical and Mechanical Treatment of Peripheral Nerves. Philadelphia, W.B. Saunders, 1922.
40. Strange, F.G. St. Clair: An Operation for Nerve Pedicle Grafting. Brit. J. Surg., *34:*423–425, 1947.
41. Strange, F.G. St. Clair: Case Report on Pedicle Nerve-Graft. Brit. J. Surg., *37:*331–333, 1950.
42. Tarlov, I.M.: Plasma Clot Suture of Peripheral Nerves and Nerve Roots. Springfield, Charles C Thomas, 1950.
43. Taylor, G.I., and Ham, F.J.: The Free Vascularized Nerve Graft. Plast. Reconstr. Surg., *57:*413–426, 1976.
44. Tsuge, K., Ikuta, Y., and Sakaue, M.: A New Technique for Nerve Suture. The Anchoring Funiculur Suture. Plast. Reconstr. Surg., *56:*496–500, 1975.
45. Williams, N.B., and Terzis, J.K.: Single Fascicular Recordings. An Intraoperative Diagnostic Tool for the Management of Peripheral Nerve Lesions. Plast. Reconstr. Surg., *57:*562–569, 1976.
46. Wrede, L.: Nervenverlagerung zur Erzwingung einer direkten Nervennaht. Zentralbl. f. Chir., *43:*529–534, 1916.
47. Young, J.Z., and Medawar, P.B.: Fibrin Suture of Peripheral Nerves. Lancet, *2:*126–128, 1940.

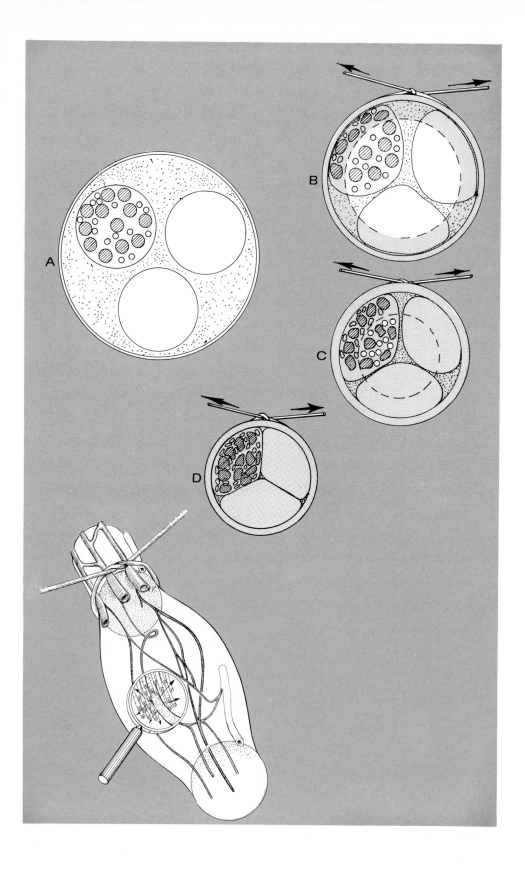

Section IV

CURRENT CONCEPT OF THE MANAGEMENT OF NERVE COMPRESSION LESIONS

CURRENT CONCEPT OF THE MANAGEMENT OF NERVE COMPRESSION LESIONS

It is the peripheral axons within a compressed nerve that suffer the greatest injury. The central fibers may be spared completely (Fig. 4 *A* and *B*). As the compression continues or increases, the central fibers become involved as well. In this central region the more heavily myelinated fibers, the motor, proprioceptive, light touch, and vibratory sensory axons are more vulnerable than the thinly myelinated, pain and sympathetic fibers (Fig. 4C). If the compression lasts long enough and is of sufficient degree, all the fibers, both sensory and motor, within the nerve are paralyzed (Fig. 4D).[21, 23, 24]

CLASSIFICATION OF NEURAL COMPRESSION LESIONS

There are two systems of classification of these neural compression lesions, one described by Sir Herbert Seddon,[19] the other by Sir Sidney Sunderland.[26] Seddon's classification utilizes the terms neurapraxia, axonotmesis and neurotmesis, while Sunderland has classified five degrees of severity of nerve injury, only the first four of which apply to compression lesions. Fifth degree nerve injury is one in which the nerve is severed and the two ends retract.

The first degree lesion of Sunderland corresponds to neurapraxia, the second degree to axonotmesis. The fourth degree, neurotmetic, lesion is a neuroma-in-continuity. There is no gross separation of the

Table 1. Correlation of Seddon and Sunderland Classification of Nerve Injury as Pertaining to Neural Compression Lesions

SEDDON	SUNDERLAND
Neurapraxia	First degree
Axonotmesis	Second degree
	Third degree
Neurotmesis	Fourth degree

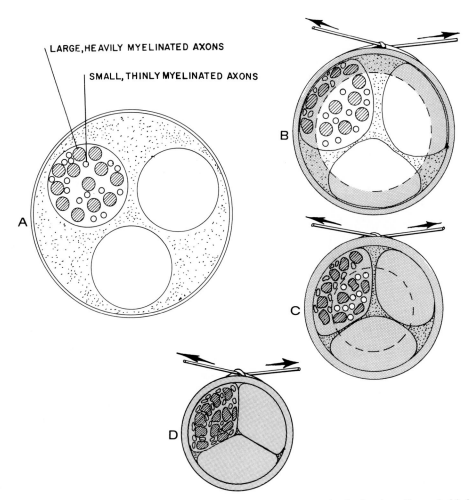

Figure 4. *A,* A multifunicular nerve is compressed in *B;* both the heavily and thinly myelinated axons in the shaded zone immediately under the epineurium lose their function. The central area axons are preserved. *C,* With increased compression the heavily myelinated axons within the central area also lose their function—only the small axons are preserved. *D,* With sufficient compression all axons cease functioning.

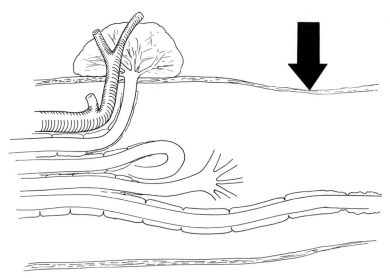

Figure 5.   With sufficient neural compression the axons become markedly disorganized and a neuroma in continuity develops. Some of the axons grow out with the blood vessels through the epineurium—forming a lateral neuroma. Others turn on themselves within the epineurium and grow proximally; while others sprout in an attempt to find and grow into the distal endoneural tubes. A few axons may be spared or may remyelinate and may be found in the distal segment of the nerve. These few axons can produce a positive Tinel sign on percussing the course of the nerve distal to the compression. With advanced localized nerve damage a Tinel sign may be present distally but, even with the lapse of time, there is no neural functional recovery when a fourth degree lesion is present. Therefore, a progressing Tinel sign may not be reliably prognostic, especially when there is failure of recovery of the proximal muscles.

nerve or retraction of nerve ends. However, the axons are in complete disarray (Fig. 5) and are not structurally in continuity.

In the third degree lesion of Sunderland, there are varying degrees of intrafunicular fibrosis. Some of these lesions are reversible and fall into the axonotmetic group. Others, in the more severe segment of third degree lesions, are irreversible because of the large number of axons involved and the extent of the irreversible fibrotic process within the funiculi.

CLINICAL CORRELATION OF THE DEGREE OF NERVE INJURY

Lesions of Neurapraxia

There appear to be three lesions of neurapraxia. The first probably is ionic and is related to electrolyte imbalance,[10] with potassium, sodium

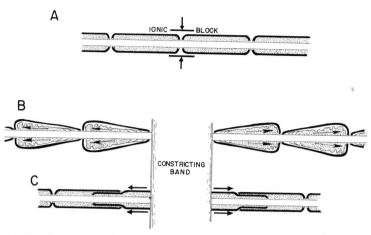

Figure 6.   *A*, The ionic type of neurapractic lesion affects the axon at the node of Ranvier. *B*, The structural lesion of neurapraxia is of the bulbous myelin type or the intussusception variety, *C*.

and ATPase disturbance at the node of Ranvier (Fig. 6*A*). The second is vascular. Classically, it has been described as an ischemia.[4] In recent years this type of neurapraxia has been attributed to an anoxia at the capillary level within the funiculi caused by venous obstruction in the epineurium (Fig. 7*A* and *B*).[12, 27] The third neurapractic lesion is mechanical, with structural changes occurring in the nerve fibers as a result of compression-shear forces. There are two basic ultrastructural lesions. The first type consists of bulbous myelin lesions with segmental tapering of internodal segments (Fig. 6*B*). The other is paranodal myelin intussusception at the node of Ranvier (Fig. 6*C*).

Table 2.   Lesions of Neurapraxia

Type	*Cause*
1. Ionic	Electrolyte imbalance
2. Vascular	Anoxia due to venous obstruction in the epineurium
3. Mechanical	Structural changes due to compression-shear forces
a. Paranodal myelin intussusception at the node of Ranvier	Acute focal compression
b. Bulbous myelin lesions with segmental tapering of internodal segments	Chronic nerve entrapment

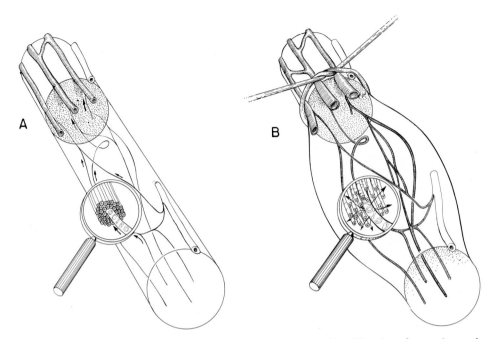

Figure 7. *A*, The circulation within the funiculus is maintained by abundant epineural, perineural, and intrafunicular circulation. There are more veins than arteries in the epineurium. *B*, With compression of the nerve, the veins in the epineurium respond to relatively minor pressure gradients resulting in increased back pressure in the capillaries at the funicular level. There are changes in the blood nerve barrier with anoxic, metabolic, and intrafunicular pressure changes which produce this type of neurapractic lesion.

It is currently believed that acute local compression produces the myelin invagination at the node of Ranvier.[7] The bulbous and tapered internodes are suspected of being the result of chronic nerve entrapment.[16]

It has been noted that both types of lesion occur away from the site of the compression.[15, 16, 17] Initially, there is segmental demyelinization, followed by healing, with segmental remyelinization. Wallerian degeneration does not occur in any neurapractic lesion. The basement membrane of the neural fiber is intact.[1]

These axon lesions have been produced in experimental animals and have been found to occur spontaneously in the guinea pig.[6] This axon-fiber pathology has been observed in man, and has been documented both in clinical entrapment lesions and in a subclinical form.[13, 14]

Clinically, the speed of return of function suggests the type of neurapractic lesion present. Rapid recovery, within hours of neurolysis, suggests the ionic or anoxic type, whereas if 30 to 60 days is necessary for recovery, the structural neurapractic lesion is most likely present.

If a patient has a persistent neural compression lesion of spontaneous or traumatic origin that lasts more than three months, surgery with exploration of the nerve at the localized level of the neural lesion is indicated. Most neurapractic lesions that respond to nonoperative measures do so within this time frame. When surgery is performed for a neurapractic lesion that has not resolved spontaneously, the response falls into two groups. In one, recovery occurs promptly, within a few hours to a few weeks after surgical intervention. The other requires about 60 days for recovery. Here, a process of demyelinization and remyelinization most likely occurs before electrical conductivity is restored. Recovery, with complete distal axonal remyelinization, would take a much longer time, as observed in wallerian degeneration and recovery with axonotmetic lesions. In contradistinction, remyelinization following wallerian degeneration usually proceeds at an average rate of 2.5 cm. per month from the site of injury to the motor end plate. It can take 5 to 6 months for a pure, complete high nerve axonotmetic lesion to regenerate to its most proximal muscle.

The typical lesions of neurapraxia may demonstrate the following clinical course.

A patient with a paralysis of the anterior interosseous branch of the median nerve of more than three months' duration at surgery, upon electrical stimulation of this branch distal to the compression, demonstrates electrical conductivity and therefore integrity of the distal axon, myelin sheath and basement membrane complex (Fig. 8). Within eight weeks after neurolysis, the patient regained volitional control of the muscles involved, the flexor pollicis longus and flexor digitorum profundus to the index and long fingers and pronator quadratus. This suggests that segmental remyelinization rather than wallerian degeneration was the mode of healing the neural lesion.

Following neurolysis of a nerve which contains predominantly sensory fibers sensibility frequently returns rapidly. Within hours of release of an entrapped digital nerve a patient can have sensation restored in the specific autonomous area.

A question that almost always occurs is: When should a neurapractic lesion require neurolysis? If the patient has electrical and clinical evidence of failure to recover sensory or motor function within a time frame of three months, then surgery is indicated. If left untreated, a neurapractic lesion of a nerve segment can increase in its degree of severity. Thus, a neurolysis of a high neural lesion, either at the elbow or the arm, can be followed by prompt return of sensation if the lesion is of the ionic or anoxic type. Approximately sixty days is necessary for recovery if the nerve fiber neurapractic lesion is of the local segmental intussusception type which requires local demyelinization and remyelinization. In this neurapractic lesion the level of the lesion plays no part in the recovery,

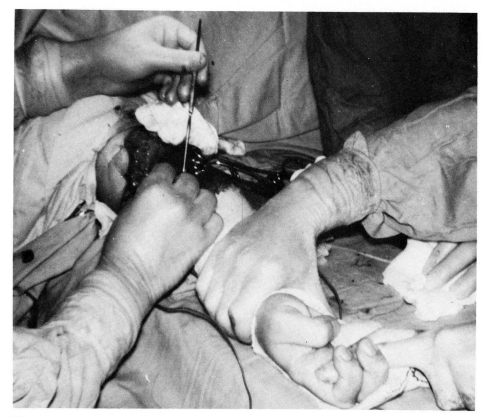

Figure 8.   The patient clinically had a complete anterior interosseous nerve paralysis. Electrical stimulation of this motor branch distal to the compression produced flexion of the terminal phalanx of the thumb, index, and long fingers. This indicated that a neurapractic lesion was present and the distal axon structure was intact.

for as soon as the remyelinization of the segmental lesion occurs electrical function is restored. Thus, it would take 60 days for neural recovery whether this structural neurapractic lesion is at the level of the axilla or 2.5 cm. from the end plate of the muscle or sensory end organ.

It has been said in the past that, if recovery of neural function following neurolysis occurs within two months, then regeneration was probably under way prior to the surgery and perhaps the neurolysis was unnecessary. With these new ultrastructural observations of the segmental neurapractic lesion,[15] one must reappraise the significance of nerve recovery 60 days after neurolysis. This period may well represent the time necessary for healing of the segmental neurapractic lesion. This would further support the need for surgical intervention if the timetable for spontaneous nerve recovery has exceeded its expected schedule.

Axonotmetic Compression Lesions

In Sunderland's classification all second degree and mild third degree lesions fall within the category of axonotmetic compression lesions. With the mild third degree lesion there is some intrafunicular fibrosis. The nerve fiber afflicted with a pure axonotmetic lesion is physiologically severed at the point of the compression. However, the basement membrane of the axon is maintained. Nevertheless, there is complete wallerian degeneration distal to the level of the compression. In the healing process new axonal sprouting and growth must occur distally from the point of axon disruption. The axon must regrow and the myelin sheath must be re-formed from this point. Actually the axonal regeneration commences one node of Ranvier proximal to the neural lesion, or a few nodes away, depending on the severity of the injury.

The recovery period in a pure axonotmetic lesion depends on the proximity of the motor end plates and sensory end organs. The more proximal the motor end plates, the earlier the recovery. The recovery takes place in a sequential pattern depending on the distance from the point of compression to the point of renervation of the muscle fiber or sensory end organ.

Classically, regeneration occurs at the rate of one millimeter per day. Axonotmetic neural lesions may heal at a more rapid rate because the basement membranes of the neural tubes are intact.

Neurotmetic Compression Lesions

This group is composed of all fourth degree Sunderland nerve lesions and includes the advanced third degree lesion. In the fourth degree lesion there is complete fibrosis of a segment of the nerve. The internal architecture of the funiculi is severely altered. A lateral neuroma may be present. With a complete neurotmetic lesion a nonfunctioning, nonconductive neuroma-in-continuity is present.

Advanced third degree lesions with extensive internal fibrosis also must be considered in this group and must be treated accordingly.

With a neurotmetic lesion, excision of the neuroma and repair is indicated. This can be achieved best by epineural repair. If the gap is too great for direct approximation, interfunicular grafting is necessary. Other appropriate techniques for overcoming nerve gaps can also be considered.

The prognosis for motor recovery following nerve repair is poor if paralysis has been complete, clinically and electrically, for more than 10 to 15 months. Successful recovery following neurorrhaphy in these cases depends on the specific nerve involved, the duration of the paralysis, the age of the patient and the level of the complete neurotmetic lesion. Neurorrhaphy is least successful for high ulnar nerve complete lesions. There is little hope for ulnar nerve recovery at this level if more than 10 months has elapsed. In contradistinction, low median nerve complete lesions can recover following repair well beyond this period. Primary muscle transfers may be the procedure of choice when the total paralysis extends beyond this critical time period.

Sensory recovery differs. Following nerve repair, essential sensory restoration has been achieved beyond this period. Success has been reported with a 25-year-old neurotmetic lesion.

FACTORS AFFECTING RETURN OF FUNCTION OF NERVE COMPRESSION LESIONS

The most important factor affecting return of function in nerve compression lesions is the nerve fiber pathology. Other factors are the level of the lesion, the duration of the compression, the status of the denervated muscles and sensory end organs, hereditary predisposition and multiple compression sites.

Eighteen months of continuous total paralysis is the limit beyond which one would not expect neural recovery. In this instance, tendon transfer would be indicated primarily. With such prolonged denervation the afflicted muscles initially atrophy and subsequently become fibrotic. However, there is evidence that some sensory end organs survive a much longer period. If the paralysis is not complete, neurolysis should be performed even beyond this 18-month period.

The advanced age of a patient is not a factor in prognosis for return of neuromuscular function in this group of cases.[11]

Hereditary factors do exist. Families and isolated cases have been reported in which the patient's nerves were pressure-sensitive. Recurrent episodes and multiple peripheral nerve involvement have been reported.[1, 5, 8] Axonal structural changes have been described. Very little is known about the hereditary mechanism which predisposes the patient to these lesions. Whether underlying chromosomal and enzymatic factors exist is strictly hypothetical at this time.

A peripheral nerve can, in its passage through the arm, be compressed at more than one level. The term "double crush" nerve-entrapment has been applied to this concept.[28] Improvement in the symptoms can be achieved with release of one of the multiple sites. On occasion treatment directed to other sites of the nerve may be necessary.

MANAGEMENT OF NERVE COMPRESSION LESIONS

Only by evaluating the entire case — the history, the clinical findings, the duration and the age of the patient, along with the operative findings — can one determine the extent of the surgical treatment necessary to restore function in nerve compression lesions. If there is failure to achieve expected recovery of neural function, surgical intervention should be planned.

Neural compression lesions that can be defined with certainty as first, second, third or fourth degree lesions are rare. They are most often mixed. One can differentiate the degree and extent of each lesion by serial clinical examinations. A fiber dissociation in compression lesions is a good prognostic sign. Prompt recovery can follow release. The large myelinated fibers (motor and proprioceptive, light touch and vibratory fibers) are more sensitive to compression. My experience with partial lesions has been rewarding following appropriately timed surgery.

If there has not been progressive improvement in function, generally by three to four months, surgery is indicated for compression lesions.

There are well-known and well-described neural compression lesions of the upper extremity which present with distinct syndromes. Examples are the carpal tunnel, Guyon's tunnel, pronator and cubital tunnel syndromes. The localization of the lesion should be confirmed by electrical testing. On occasion, anatomical variations or variant clinical patterns such as Sudeck's atrophy[25] in association with a nerve entrapment can cloud the problem. It is essential, therefore, that the level of the neural compression be located accurately. For example, if the patient has a high median nerve lesion, decompression at the wrist will not relieve the patient's symptoms. In order to successfully manage a nerve entrapment lesion accurate diagnosis and localization of the pathologic process is essential.

Only with careful anatomical exposure, initially of the gross neural structure and subsequently of the fine internal structure in normal neural tissue proximal and distal to the lesion, can one properly evaluate the pathology. In this manner one can avoid inadvertent conversion of a second degree Sunderland lesion to a fifth degree lesion, in which the nerve is severed and the ends retract.

The extent of the anatomical exposure is always much greater than the size of the neural lesion would at first suggest. For example, if the lesion is an inch long, surgical incision at least five inches long is necessary. Particular care must be taken to avoid injury to the superficial skin nerves when surgery is necessary for this group of patients. Postoperative symptomatic neuromata of skin nerves can be a major complication. The neural structure is identified grossly in the normal tissue proximal and distal to its entrapment. From both the proximal and distal sides, the dissection proceeds, separating the epineurium from its scarred bed. As one approaches the area of maximum entrapment, if there is a fibrotic band, suddenly with release of this offending structure the entire nerve is liberated. There may be a small residual area of indentation in the nerve. With an intraneural injection of saline one can observe the ease of flow. If there is any obstruction, a localized neurolysis is necessary.

The neurolysis most often separates the epineurium from its scarred bed or removes crossing thrombosed vessels or thickened fascia, but on occasion the funiculi may require internal dissection.[3, 18]

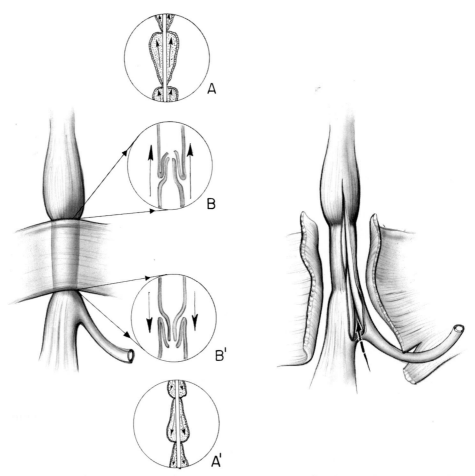

Figure 9.   Some carpal tunnel release procedures require internal neurolysis of the median nerve. When thenar atrophy is the predominant clinical finding, neurolysis of the motor branch through the flexor retinaculum is performed if the recurrent motor branch has a transligamentous course. In addition, the motor funiculi are liberated at the proximal and distal levels of the retinaculum where the compression is usually most marked (diagram on right). Insert A-A' and B-B' depict on an axon level the direction and the type myelin deformities seen with the mechanical lesion of neurapraxia.

When I include an internal neurolysis, I correlate it strictly with the patient's symptoms. For example, in a carpal tunnel syndrome with advanced thenar atrophy and minimal sensory disturbance, after release of the flexor retinaculum, the motor branch is identified and is traced from its origin at the median nerve distally into the thenar muscles. In this distal course it frequently penetrates a separate foramen in the flexor retinaculum which may be the offending obstructive site. The compression may occur at the proximal or distal level of this retinaculum. In Figure 9 this motor funiculus is traced proximally through the main median nerve trunk, including the area distal and proximal to the edges of the flexor retinaculum. Frequently in the carpal tunnel syndrome pain and numbness are the major factors. Very often the long finger is most involved. In these cases, after opening the epineurium, the medial two or three funiculi are separated, commencing distally and then working proximally through the region in the median nerve covered by the edges of the flexor retinaculum, leaving the other funiculi untraumatized. I do not perform any internal neurolysis which involves all the funiculi of the median nerve in a carpal tunnel syndrome. In elderly patients, long finger discomfort and dysesthesias persist long after isolated carpal tunnel release. By including selective internal neurolysis in patients operated for this syndrome where long finger pain predominates preoperatively, this morbidity has been improved markedly.

Internal neurolysis when utilized should be adapted to the individual case. It should be limited to those fasciculi that are clinically involved. Extensive internal neurolysis can induce fibrosis in all layers of the nerve.[18] The perineurium should be violated only on rare occasions, with specific indications, as, for example, when the patient has a third degree lesion with intraneural fibrosis. The degree of the internal fibrosis and thus the extent of the third degree lesion within the nerve may not be clear. Therefore, the perineurium may be opened in selected cases. The integrity of the perineurium is important for normal neural function. It acts as a supporting structure for maintenance of a normal elevated pressure within the funiculus. Furthermore, it maintains the milieu within the funiculus. It acts as a barrier for the passage of proteins and other large molecules.

When the perineurium is violated there is a herniation of axons. The axons that bulge out of the perineurial window demonstrate pathological changes. Initially, there is segmental demyelinization. This is followed by localized remyelinization, with restoration of the perineurium.[22] In clinical cases in which pain is due to a localized neural lesion, the epineurium is frequently opened, but the perineurium rarely.

Intraoperative evaluation of the funiculi is best achieved with the single fascicular recording technique.[29] Furthermore, correlating the clinical preoperative assessment with operative findings of firmness of individual funiculi palpated with the aid of the scalpel handle can be helpful in localizing and deciding which funiculus is to be opened. The operating room microscope is an important adjunct in further evaluating the funiculus by direct magnified inspection and in the technique of opening the perineurium.

The neurotmetic lesions — the far advanced third and fourth degree lesions — require special care in their evaluation.

EVALUATION OF THE NEUROMA-IN-CONTINUITY

There are several ways one can evaluate a neuroma-in-continuity. Once it has been established that surgery is indicated, since there is not going to be spontaneous recovery, intraoperative techniques are used to evaluate the neural lesion. At surgery electrical stimulation proximal and distal to the neuroma prior to freeing it completely, with direct observation of the peripheral muscle and limb response, is useful.[20, 26] More refined intraoperative conduction studies across the neuroma are valuable but require more sophisticated instrumentation.[9, 29] If the neuroma is stony hard to palpation proximal to the compression, then the prognosis is poor for neural recovery by neurolysis alone. Conversely, a soft enlargement of the nerve is a favorable surgical observation for restoration of neural function. Furthermore, intraneural saline injection followed by external and internal neurolysis as necessary, utilizing the operating microscope or ocular magnification, can be helpful in these cases.[2] Thus, if the neuroma is stony hard and a spontaneous neural lesion has existed for about 18 months, then recovery by neurolysis, nerve excision and nerve repair or grafting is not likely. However, if the lesion has been partial even beyond an 18-month period, then recovery can occur following external and internal neurolysis techniques alone. The important clinical factor is the duration of the complete paralysis.

Finally, further evaluation with new tools and techniques, such as the determination of intrafunicular pressure and the development of neurotrophic substances, can be expected to bring additional knowledge to this field. By keeping aware of these new scientific advances we can increase our understanding of these neural problems and ultimately increase our effectiveness in the care of our patients.

BIBLIOGRAPHY

1. Behse, F., Buchthal, F., Carlsen, F., and Knappeis, G.G.: Hereditary Neuropathy with Liability to Pressure Palsies: Electrophysiological and Histopathological Aspects. Brain, 95:777–794, 1972.
2. Brown, B.A.: Internal Neurolysis in Traumatic Peripheral Nerve Lesions in Continuity. Surg. Clin. N. Am., 52:1167–1175, 1972.

 3. Curtis, R.M. and Eversmann, W.W.: Internal Neurolysis as an Adjunct to the Treatment of the Carpal-Tunnel Syndrome. J. Bone Joint Surg., *55A*:733–740, 1973.
 4. Denny-Brown, D., and Brenner, C.: Paralysis of Nerve Induced by Direct Pressure and by Tourniquet. Arch. Neurol. Psychiat., *51*:1–26, 1944.
 5. Earl, C.J., Fullerton, P.M., Wakefield, G.S., and Schutta, H.S.: Hereditary Neuropathy with Liability to Pressure Palsies. A Clinical and Electrophysiological Study of Four Families. Quart. J. Med., *33*:481–498, 1964.
 6. Fullerton, P.M., and Gilliatt, R.W.: Pressure Neuropathy in the Hindfoot of the Guinea Pig. J. Neurol. Neurosurg. Psychiat., *30*:18–25, 1967.
 7. Gilliatt, R.W., Ochoa, J., Rudge, P., and Neary, D.: The Cause of Nerve Damage in Acute Compression. Trans. Am. Neurol. Assoc., *99*:71–74, 1974.
 8. Karpati, G., Carpenter, S., Eisen, A.A., and Feindel, W.: Familial Multiple Peripheral Nerve Entrapments—An Unusual Manifestation of a Peripheral Neuropathy. Trans. Am. Neurol. Assoc., *98*:267–269, 1973.
 9. Kline, D.G., and Nulsen, F.E.: The Neuroma in Continuity. Its Preoperative and Operative Management. Surg. Clin. N. Am., *52*:1189–1209, 1972.
10. Kuczynski, K.: Functional Micro-anatomy of the Peripheral Nerve Trunks. Hand, *6*:1–10, 1974.
11. Levine, J., and Spinner, M.: Neurolysis in Elderly Patients. Clin. Orthop., *80*:13–16, 1971.
12. Lundborg, G.: Ischemic Nerve Injury. Experimental Studies on Intraneural Microvascular Pathophysiology and Nerve Function in a Limb Subjected to Temporary Circulatory Arrest. Scand. J. Plast. Reconstr. Surg., Suppl. 6, 1–113, 1970.
13. Neary, D., and Eames, R.A.: The Pathology of Ulnar Nerve Compression in Man. Neuropathol. Appl. Neurobiol., *1*:69–88, 1975.
14. Neary, D., Ochoa, J., and Gilliatt, R.W.: Subclinical Entrapment Neuropathy in Man. J. Neurol. Sci., *24*:283–298, 1976.
15. Ochoa, J., Fowler, T.J., and Gilliatt, R.W.: Anatomical Changes in Peripheral Nerves Compressed by Pneumatic Tourniquet. J. Anat., *113*:433–455, 1972.
16. Ochoa, J.: Schwann Cell and Myelin Changes Caused by some Toxic Agents and Trauma. Proc. Roy. Soc. Med., *67*:3–4, 1974.
17. Rudge, P., Ochoa, J., and Gilliatt, R.W.: Acute Peripheral Nerve Compression in the Baboon. J. Neurol. Sci., *23*:403–420, 1974.
18. Rydevik, B., Lundborg, G., and Nordborg, C.: Intraneural Tissue Reactions Induced by Internal Neurolysis. Scand. J. Plast. Reconstr. Surg., *10*:3–8, 1976.
19. Seddon, H.J.: Three Types of Nerve Injury. Brain, *66*:237–288, 1943.
20. Seddon, H.J.: Surgical Disorders of the Peripheral Nerves. Second edition, Edinburgh, Churchill Livingstone, 1975.
21. Spencer, P.S.: Light and Electron Microscopic Observations on Localized Peripheral Nerve Injuries. Thesis, 2 vols. London, University of London, 1971.
22. Spencer, P.S., Weinberg, H., Raine, C.S., and Prineas, J.W.: The Perineurial Window—A New Model of Focal Demyelination and Remyelination. Brain Res., *96*:323–329, 1975.
23. Spinner, M.: Compression Nerve Injuries. *In* Symposium on Microsurgery, Educational Foundation of the American Society of Plastic and Reconstructive Surgeons. A.I. Daniller, and B. Strauch (eds.), St. Louis, The C.V. Mosby Co., 1976, Vol. 14, pp. 161–171.
24. Spinner, M., and Spencer, P.S.: Nerve Compression Lesions of the Upper Extremity. A Clinical and Experimental Review. Clin. Orthop., *104*:46–67, 1974.
25. Stein, A.H. Jr.: The Relation of Median Nerve Compression to Sudeck's Syndrome. Surg. Gynecol. Obstet., *115*:713–720, 1962.
26. Sunderland, S.: Nerves and Nerve Injuries. Baltimore, Williams & Wilkins, 1968.
27. Sunderland, S.: Nerve Lesion in the Carpal Tunnel Syndrome. J. Neurol. Neurosurg. Psychiat., *39*:615–626, 1976.
28. Upton, A.R.M., and McComas, A.J.: The Double Crush in Nerve-Entrapment Syndromes. Lancet, *2*:359–362, 1973.
29. Williams, H.B., and Terzis, J.K.: Single Fascicular Recordings: An Intraoperative Diagnostic Tool for the Management of Peripheral Nerve Lesions. Plast. Reconstr. Surg., *57*:562–569, 1976.

FACTORS AFFECTING RETURN OF FUNCTION FOLLOWING NERVE INJURY

FACTORS AFFECTING RETURN OF FUNCTION FOLLOWING NERVE INJURY

＊The factors which affect the end result of injury to a peripheral nerve or its branches include the following: the age of the patient, the type of repair, the type of injury to the nerve, the level of the injury, the length of time from injury to repair, the tension at the suture line, the length of the nerve gap, the vascular supply to the nerve, the presence of open distal axon tubes, the bed for the repair, the overall nutrition of the extremity, and infection. Many of these factors are interrelated, for example, the technique for the repair, the patency of the axon tubes, and the tension at the suture line.

Critical evaluation of the sensory, motor, and autonomic recovery following nerve repair is vital in determining these factors.[13] One must have knowledge of the numerous variant communicating neural pathways, of dual innervation of muscles, and of the trick motions that patients with isolated muscle paralysis develop to compensate for the functional loss before the neural recovery can be truly assessed. Results of the repair of complete and partial nerve lesions cannot be evaluated together. Partial lesions have an area of neurapraxia within the intact portion of the nerve adjacent to the lacerated fibers.[5] Following neurorrhaphy, early recovery is due to the resolution of the first degree component of the lesion rather than to the excellence of the repair of the fifth degree portion of the neural lesion.

Of all the factors affecting the return of neural function following complete neural injury, the age of the patient, the type of injury to the nerve, the technique, and the timing of the repair are the main influences affecting the return of function. The contemporary technique of nerve repair has been discussed in the preceding chapter.

AGE. Souttar,[17] Bowden,[2] Lindsay, Walker, and Farmer,[7] and Sakellarides,[15] have clearly documented the excellent results, both sensory and motor, of nerve surgery in the child and adolescent. Even complete ulnar nerve injuries, which have the poorest prognosis in the adult, can be expected to recover more readily in the child. Lindsay et al.[7] have noted that in their group of children with ulnar nerve repair the most common disability was weakness in adduction of the little finger. In a review of my cases I have occasionally noted similar residual paresis of the third palmar interosseous muscle in children, with a more common occurrence in adults. It should be noted that even mixed nerves seem to respond to repair better in children. In addition, the rate of return of function is more rapid for the child than for the adult. It is not only the smaller size of the limb which accounts for this but also the increased actual rate of axon regeneration. When eliciting the Tinel sign in children, I have been impressed by the rapid advance of the sign and its early disappearance (much earlier than in adults). The residual pain frequently observed in adults on percussion at the site of suture repair is rarely observed in the younger group. The precise reason for this clinical observation of the influence of age on the end result in neurorrhaphy is not fully understood at the present time. It has been suggested that the child's central nervous system has a greater capability to adapt than the adult's, thus resulting in alleged better response to peripheral nerve repair.

TYPE OF INJURY. The type of injury affects the prognosis. For example, an ice-pick injury to a nerve is certainly different from a military injury caused by an M16 rifle bullet. Similarly, the soft tissue damage caused by a .22 caliber rifle bullet is usually much less than that caused by shotgun pellets and wadding.

Likewise, as a group, lesions in continuity that result from civilian injury offer a different prognosis and should be treated differently from military injuries. An excellent description of the lesion in military wounds, and its prognosis, with the often found extensive intraneural fibrosis and partial lateral neuromas of the nerve, has been presented by Zachary and Roaf.[21] They were of the opinion that neurolysis was of little use in the treatment of lesions in continuity. Bateman,[1] however, as a result of his study on civilian nerve injury, found that neurolysis was extremely valuable in treating this group of lesions. My experience supports Bateman's view.

In injuries caused by low velocity missiles the prognosis is usually better than in high velocity injuries, especially if the nerve palsy is delayed in onset. In tight compartment areas, such as the carpal tunnel, Guyon's tunnel, and the cubital tunnel, the swelling within the restraining compartment should be relieved early to obtain maximum recovery in the shortest time. In civilian, low velocity bullet injuries, in which no tight compartment exists in the pathway, I have elected to treat the nerve lesion by secondary repair, if necessary, because the majority have recovered spontaneously.

External compressive lesions, whether at the carpal tunnel or at one of the other sites in the arm, respond well as a group to neurolysis, provided the paralysis has not extended beyond the irreversible period of muscle degeneration (12 to 18 months). In addition, scar entrapment of nerves shows a similarly favorable response.

When a fourth or fifth degree neural lesion is high in the extremity, the prognosis for excellent recovery following repair is unlikely because of several factors. Proximally, there is a greater mixture of sensory and motor funiculi, and it is harder to restore the usual sensory and motor alignment. In addition, the closer the injury is to the cell body, the more frequently death of the cell body itself occurs. Thus, without a cell body, regeneration of the axon cannot occur.

Electrical injuries are known to cause marked local fibrosis. They too can produce profound central death of cells in the proximal sensory ganglions and within the anterior motor horn cells. The prognosis for the quality of peripheral nerve regeneration following nerve repair is guarded. It is adversely affected by the severity of the electrical damage.

Crush injuries and contusions of the nerves following a direct blow or fracture have a much better overall prognosis of recovery than do other nerve injuries. The statistics improve when the group of cases in which the nerve is entrapped in bone fragments is recognized early. Most nerve injuries associated with closed fractures or dislocation will recover spontaneously after reduction. Statistically, when surgical intervention is specifically indicated neurolysis appears to produce an excellent recovery rate for this group of injuries. If a nerve does not demonstrate clinical or electromyographic evidence of recovery by four months following fracture or dislocation, exploration of the neural injury is indicated.

It has been said by some authors that perhaps if one had waited longer the nerve would have recovered by itself. However, there is a definite place for external neurolysis, with or without incision of the epineurium. Leonard,[6] in five cases, has shown immediate improvement of sensation following release of extraneural compression. Similarly, in my own experience I have seen sensation return to a hypoesthetic or anesthetic area immediately after surgery.

Motor recovery following neurolysis often follows an axonotmetic pattern. The first muscle to be reinnervated is the one whose end-plates are closest to the point of nerve compression. Thus the shorter the distance through which regeneration must occur, the earlier the return of function can be expected. Similarly, within a compressed nerve with mixed motor and sensory fibers, I have seen a neurapractic lesion in one fascicle and an axonotmetic lesion in an adjacent funiculus. Often the sensory funicular lesion is neurapractic, and its function returns promptly.

A peripheral nerve lesion that produces at the time of injury a dissociated paralysis has a better prognosis for spontaneous recovery than does one that produces a complete paralysis.[18] Heavily myelinated axons are more affected by trauma than are thinner ones. The motor fibers and some of the sensory fibers are heavily myelinated. When motor paralysis is present out of proportion to the sensory disturbance, the prognosis is usually favorable. However, the examining physician must be certain that the clinical pattern of motor loss is not typical of that seen with pure posterior interosseous nerve paralysis, anterior interosseous nerve paralysis or isolated paralysis involving the deep branch of the ulnar nerve. In this latter group, there are no sensory abnormalities, while with a dissociated neural lesion of a main peripheral nerve there are sensory disturbances involving proprioception, vibration, pressure, and touch but the thinly myelinated pain, temperature, and autonomic fibers are preserved.[9] A patient who has motor paralysis and responds to pin prick (pain) is not hysterical; he probably has a dissociated peripheral nerve lesion with a good prognosis. This can be confirmed by further sensory differential testing.

TIMING OF NERVE REPAIR.   There is a difference of opinion concerning primary and secondary repair of severed nerves in civilian injuries. The English school, led by Nicholson and Seddon[11] and Zachary and Holmes,[20] are proponents of secondary repair. American writers Boyes,[3] Milford,[8] Nichols,[10] and Grabb[4] are proponents of primary repair. The Australians, Rank, Wakefield, and Hueston,[14] on the basis of their studies, support primary repair. My own experience favors primary repair. There seems to be very little controversy concerning the need for secondary repair when dealing with military nerve injuries, with civilian and industrial nerve injuries that are dirty and severely traumatized, and with civilian gunshot lesions.

Recently, the concept of delayed primary repair of peripheral nerves has been suggested, the repair being performed on the fifth to tenth day after debridement and closure. I have utilized this repair sequence only in specific instances; for example, when other concurrent major injuries to the abdomen or thorax preclude primary nerve repair in the forearm. Circumstances can improve rapidly, permitting delayed primary repair (Fig. 84). Had other injuries not been present the nerve lesion would have been ideal for primary repair. On occasion, wounds of the forearm, such as those caused by the fan of an automobile engine, demand initial debridement and closure if possible. If the wound becomes sound and the initial culture is sterile, delayed primary repair on the fifth to tenth day may be successfully performed; however, it must be stressed that the dissection is more difficult and that gentleness in surgical tissue handling is demanded in order to avoid excessive scarring about the tendons and repaired nerves. The delayed primary repair technique should not be a routine nerve repair procedure. It should be reserved for specific situations and should only be employed by those experienced in all aspects of the method.

Partial nerve injuries are best repaired primarily (Fig. 10). In the scarring seen at 3 weeks it often is difficult to fully evaluate which nerve bundles are involved and which are clear. For example, a 36-year-old man had a laceration of the median nerve with almost total sensory loss in the

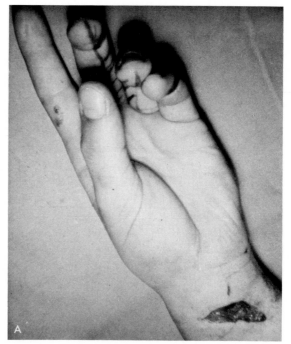

Figure 10.   *A*, Partial median nerve injury is evident. Sensation is absent only in the third cleft. Normal opposition of the thumb is present.

Illustration continued on opposite page.

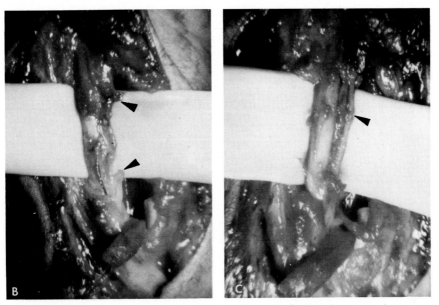

Figure 10 *Continued.*   B, There is a laceration of one funiculus, the two ends (arrows) of which are seen ulnarly on the Penrose drain. C, The funiculus is repaired primarily (arrow), accurately and with technical ease.

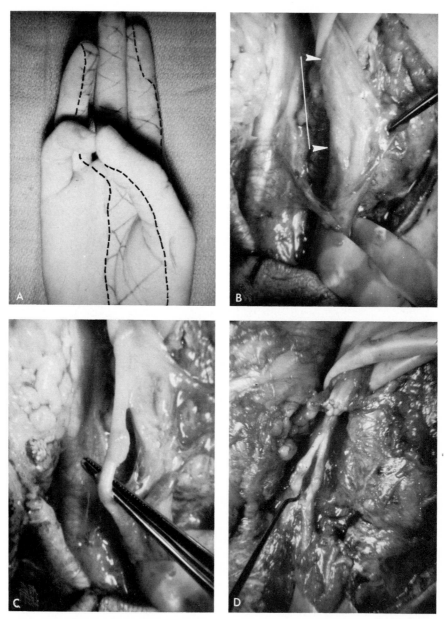

Figure 11.   *A*, The right hand reveals full opposition of the thumb. Sensation is absent in the median distribution of the hand except for a small area on the radial side of the pulp of the index finger. *B*, The scarred median nerve (bracketed arrows) is noted with the epineurium incised. The funicular pattern is markedly disturbed. *C* and *D*, Under the dissecting microscope each funiculus was identified. Firm small neuromata were found in all except for a portion of one. The anomalous innervation of the entire thenar muscles was from the ulnar nerve.

median innervated 3½ fingers. Yet there was normal opposition of the thumb (Fig. 11A). With care the funiculi with their neuromata could be identified (Fig. 11B–D). Certainly primary repair in partial nerve injuries of varying degrees is technically easier and produces the most rewarding results.

To evaluate the return of motor function, the anastomotic pathways in the hand and forearm must be eliminated in order to determine the true return of motor function of a severed nerve. Overlap of a sensory nerve must also be considered in evaluating a return of sensory function.

Statistics must be defined not only in terms of success or failure but also in relation to the nature of the lesion and the presence or absence of associated soft tissue injuries. Each peripheral nerve of the forearm in an adult has a distinct prognostic pattern. It is well known that recovery in the ulnar nerve is not as good as in the median and the radial nerves. Likewise the radial nerve has a better recovery rate than the median nerve.

In the forearm, another important factor affecting the end result is the fact that for many of the branches, the distance from the level of the laceration or entrapment to the point of reinnervation is short, so there is a strong argument to be made for primary repairs of the major branches of the peripheral nerves of the forearm. Sometimes the length of regeneration from the point of severance to the muscle belly may only be 5 to 7 cm. Of course war wounds in which massive destruction of soft tissue has occurred, as noted during the conflicts of this century, certainly end up with a higher failure rate than civilian injuries. Seddon[16] noted that 20 per cent of 699 World War II nerve injuries were too extensive to be repaired.

Nicholson and Seddon[11] reported that in a civilian population (305 median and ulnar nerve lesions) 65 per cent of the low median nerves regained useful motor function and 79 per cent regained useful sensory function. The wartime study of Zachary[19] (covering more than 670 median and ulnar nerve lesions) revealed useful return of motor function in 42 per cent and useful sensory function in 68 per cent. As regards the low ulnar lesion in the civilian group, 82 per cent regained useful motor and sensory function and 35 per cent obtained some independent lateral movement, compared to a 78 per cent return of useful motor activity and 65 per cent useful sensory function, with 16 per cent regaining independent lateral movement in the instances of military injury.

Omer[12] found (in a study of 917 upper extremity neural lesions sustained during the Vietnam war) that when the nerve remained in continuity, spontaneous recovery occurred in 70 per cent of gunshot wounds and in 85 per cent of fractures and dislocations. It took 3 to 9 months for gunshot injuries to recover, whereas recovery from fractures occurred in 1 to 4 months. When the nerves were severed, epineurial repair was successful in 44 per cent of lacerations and 25 per cent of gunshot wounds.

The 670 personal cases of nerve injury reviewed for this study must be analyzed carefully in order that the proper conclusions be drawn. Of this group of cases 45 per cent must be excluded from serious analysis because of lack of adequate long term (5 year) followup. The greater portion of cases excluded are from the military service (American and Korean soldiers) and from city hospitals where changes of address are rapid, with people moving out of the state and, at times, out of the country. The remaining 390 cases, drawn from my private practice and from the previously mentioned group, support the following conclusions:

1. Children have an excellent prognosis for return of sensory and motor function (43 of 46 cases) following nerve severance and repair.

2. If an entrapped peripheral nerve or its major branch is released before irreversible muscle damage has occurred, then the results are excellent (170 of 175 cases).

3. The results of the remaining 169 cases in this series support the concept of primary repair of partial and complete nerve injuries in the usual type of civilian injury.

In summary, it is generally agreed that the younger the patient the better the prognosis for the completeness and the rate of recovery. It also appears evident that the value placed on the technique of neurolysis and scar removal depends on whether the clinician has been evaluating civilian or military injuries. In civilian life neurolysis in the appropriate situation appears to be a most useful modality.

BIBLIOGRAPHY

1. Bateman, J. E.: Trauma to Nerves in Limbs. Philadelphia, W. B. Saunders, 1962, p. 167.
2. Bowden, R. E. M.: Factors Influencing Functional Recovery. *In* Seddon, H. J. (Ed.): Peripheral Nerve Injuries. London, Her Majesty's Stationery Office, 1954.
3. Boyes, J. H.: Bunnell's Surgery of the Hand. Ed. 5, Philadelphia, Lippincott, 1970, p. 375.
4. Grabb, W. C.: Management of Nerve Injuries in the Forearm. Orth. Clin., *1*:2, 419–431, 1970.
5. Hudson, A. R., and Kline, D. G.: Progression of Partial Experimental Injury to Peripheral Nerve. Part 2: Light and Electron Microscopic Studies. J. Neurosurg., *42*:15–22, 1975.
6. Leonard, M. H.: Immediate Improvement of Sensation on Relief of Anoxia from Extraneural Compression. J. Bone Joint Surg., *51A*:1282–1284, 1969.
7. Lindsay, W. K., Walker, F. G., and Farmer, A. W.: Traumatic Peripheral Nerve Injuries in Children. Plast. Reconstr. Surg., *30*:462–468, 1962.
8. Milford, L.: The Hand. St. Louis, Mosby, 1971, pp. 42–43.
9. Moldaver, J.: Tourniquet Paralysis Syndrome. Arch. Surg., *68*:136–144, 1955.
10. Nichols, H. M.: Manual of Hand Injuries. Ed. 2, Chicago, Year Book Medical Publishers, 1960, p. 229.
11. Nicholson, O. R., and Seddon, H. J.: Nerve Repair in Civil Practice. Brit. Med. J., *2*:1065–1070, 1957.
12. Omer, G.: Injuries to Nerves of the Extremity. J. Bone Joint Surg., *56A*:1615–1624, 1974.

13. Omer, G., and Spinner, M.: Peripheral Nerve Testing and Suture Techniques. *In* American Academy of Orthopedic Surgeons Instructional Course Lectures, Vol 24. St. Louis, Mosby, 1975, pp. 122–143.
14. Rank, R. K., Wakefield, A. R., and Hueston, J. T.: Surgery of Repair as Applied to Hand Injuries. Ed. 3, Baltimore, Williams & Wilkins, 1968, p. 137.
15. Sakellarides, H.: A Follow-up Study of 172 Peripheral Nerve Injuries in the Upper Extremity in Civilians. J. Bone Joint Surg., *44A*:140–148, 1962.
16. Seddon, H. J.: The Use of Autogenous Grafts for the Repair of Large Gaps in Peripheral Nerves. Brit. J. Surg., *35*:151–173, 1947.
17. Souttar, H. S.: Nerve Injuries in Children. Brit. Med. J., *2*:349–350, 1945.
18. Wortis, H., Stein, M. H., and Jolliffe, N.: Fiber Dissociation in Peripheral Neuropathy. Arch. Intern. Med., *69*:222–237, 1942.
19. Zachary, R. B.: Results of Nerve Suture. *In* Seddon, H. J. (Ed.): Peripheral Nerve Injuries. London, Her Majesty's Stationery Office, 1954.
20. Zachary, R.B., and Holmes, W.: Primary Surgery of Nerves. Surg. Gynecol. Obstet., *82*:632–651, 1946.
21. Zachary, R. B., and Roaf, R.: Lesions in Continuity. *In* Seddon, H. J. (Ed.): Peripheral Nerve Injuries. London, Her Majesty's Stationery Office, 1954.

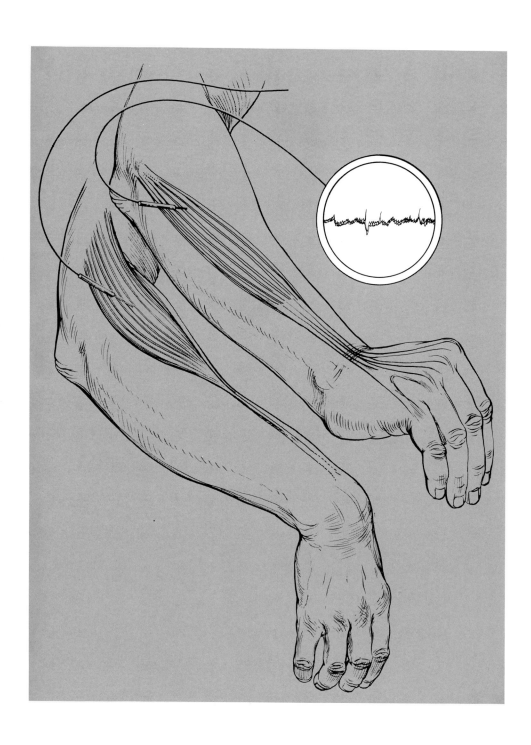

CLINICAL APPLICATIONS OF ELECTRO-NEUROMYOGRAPHIC PROCEDURES TO NEURAL LESIONS OF THE FOREARM AND HAND

CLINICAL APPLICATIONS OF ELECTRONEUROMYOGRAPHIC PROCEDURES TO NEURAL LESIONS OF THE FOREARM AND HAND

Electroneuromyographic procedures are used primarily to confirm clinical observations; they should not substitute for the reasoning processes utilized by the peripheral nerve surgeon or neurologist in arriving at the proper diagnosis. The results of electrical tests alone frequently are misleading, especially if they are viewed out of the context of the clinical aspects of a specific case.

It is often in the best interests of the patient for the peripheral nerve surgeon and the electromyographer to engage in a dialogue for the purpose of exchanging information. Specific questions can be asked, and the electromyographer can attend to these questions in the course of the examination. In a particular case the treating physician might want to know if a lesion is complete, if return of function is occurring, or if a variant nerve distribution pattern is present—as, for example, is the median nerve at the wrist carrying only sensory fibers and no motor fibers? Answers to these questions can facilitate either the accurate conservative care of the patient with a nerve lesion or encourage prompt surgery with the appropriate procedure.

Electromyographic evaluation reflects the status of a motor unit; it does not give a specific diagnosis. It can be of help in distinguishing and localizing disease processes involving muscles and nerves.[1] Information can even be obtained from the simple insertion of the needle electrode. Firmness of a muscle, for example, such as in fibrotic states of muscle associated with infection, Volkmann's disease, or longstanding denervation, may be appreciated on needle insertion.

It is vital from a clinical point of view to have some suspicion of the underlying neurological problem so that the electromyographer can sample the proper muscle or muscles to confirm a clinical diagnosis.[4, 5] Exact needle electrode placement in muscles of the forearm and hand is essential when evaluating specific injuries of major branches of peripheral nerves of the forearm. For example, in an anterior interosseous nerve paralysis, it is necessary to sample the flexor pollicis longus, the flexor digitorum profundus to the index and long fingers, and the pronator quadratus. The diagnosis is confirmed when these specific muscles are found to have a reduced interference pattern with maximal effort and a decrease of the amplitude of the evoked response.[16] Prolonged latency from the elbow to the pronator quadratus (greater than 5.1 msec.) and prolonged duration of the evoked action potential of the anterior interosseous nerve (greater than 3.6 msec.) have also been documented.[15] The remaining muscles innervated by the main median nerve trunk are usually normal, as is the sensory conductivity.

Electromyographic changes may persist 6 to 8 months after clinical recovery in an anterior interosseous nerve syndrome, while latency and duration determinations tend to return to normal values earlier, usually within 1 to 2 months.[15]

In tourniquet paralysis, similar abnormal electromyographic findings persist for half a year more after clinical recovery and return to normal of the conduction velocity.[18]

Resting normal muscle is usually electrically silent. Denervating muscle depolarizes at rest and produces spontaneous discharges, or fibrillations. The finding of fibrillations in a patient expected to have them must be accepted and considered to be of clinical significance. However, 10 per cent of patients without clinical disease have been reported to have fibrillations.[1] Similarly, 30 per cent of patients with clear-cut lower motor neuron disease do not have fibrillations.[10] Therefore, the presence or absence of fibrillations alone is not diagnostic evidence for or against a disease process. Fibrillations observed on electromyographic study must be evaluated with the entire clinical picture in mind. If the patient's clinical examination leads to a diagnosis in which fibrillations are not to be expected, these may or may not be significant and the patient may or may not have a clincal neuromuscular disease.

In evaluating a peripheral nerve problem, it is essential to determine if a short segment of the nerve or the entire length of the nerve is affected, or if multiple nerves are involved in the pathological process. When there is a segmental disturbance electromyographically, increased polyphasics occur on voluntary contraction of the muscle. The appearance of fibrillation or positive sharp waves (the term positive sharp wave should be taken in the same context and with the same implications as the term fibrillation) as well as a lack of a recruitment pattern on maximum contraction of a particular muscle is noted. Electrically, there is a conduction disturbance across the neural segment but usually not through the entire nerve.

A pure neurapractic lesion presents with a slowing of conduction across the involved segment and an absence of amplitude on voluntary effort. Electrical stimulation above the lesion does not produce an evoked response, while stimulation *below* does produce a good neuromuscular response (see Fig. 8). If the degree of nerve injury were more than first degree, that is, axonotmetic or neurotmetic with wallerian degeneration, only then would fibrillation, sharp waves, and complex potentials be observed.

To be of value, conduction velocity studies must be reproducible so that comparative values can be used in evaluating the patient's clinical progress. Conduction velocity is a measurement of the speed of conduction along a nerve. Usually both motor and sensory conductions are determined and are expressed in meters per second.

Technically, electronic instrumentation consisting of an electronic stimulator, a preamplifer, an oscilloscope, a calibration signal, an accurate time base and photographic documentation are necessary.

By recording from two points along a nerve (and, when determining motor conduction velocity, recording the initial response from the innervated distal muscle), appropriate values can be obtained. It is necessary to know the distance between the two points of stimulation in order to determine the motor conduction velocity.

Sensory conduction is determined by stimulating, distally or proximally, at two points and, depending upon which technique is utilized — antidromic or orthodromic — recording either proximally or distally. It is necessary to measure the timing of the low voltage sensory evoked potential as well as the distance between the two sites of stimuation.

Even though conduction velocity determinations along a nerve are relatively simple, easily reproducible, and dependable, errors can occur. There are numerous factors that can affect the accuracy of these determinations.

FACTORS THAT AFFECT CONDUCTION VELOCITY DETERMINATIONS

1. Temperature. The colder a room, and therefore the colder the patient, the more there is slowing of the conduction velocity. Different temperature gradients exist throughout the body. In a limb the distal temperature is lower than the proximal. Therefore, a segmental conduction velocity determination across neural segments of the proximal area would be faster than a similar determination more distally in the same limb.

2. Age. Newborns have conduction velocities approximately half those of the normal adult. Within the first 3 years the velocity increases to normal levels. Older patients also have a slower conduction velocity, in the realm of 10 per cent below the average for adults.[10]

3. In evaluating regenerating nerve fibers the electromyographer needs to utilize supramaximal stimuli or the "marble" effect results, and false conduction values are obtained.[6]

4. Technical errors, such as stimulating adjacent nerves when anomalies exist, can give false conduction values. Furthermore, if only one site rather than two is stimulated, and the distance between this electrode and the recording is determined using only one site, false or inaccurate conduction velocity values are calculated.

5. Heavy or edematous limbs can give false determinations. The site of stimuation on the skin may not be the exact point of nerve stimuation within the limb.[17]

In specific areas — for example, across the thoracic outlet — the use of a measuring tape rather than fixed calipers has been found to give unreliable conduction values. In this important area, where the physician's clinical opinion requires laboratory substantiation, use of specially adapted obstetrical calipers has been demonstrated to produce accurate and reliable conduction values.[14] Similarly, when determining conduction values of the ulnar nerve across the elbow, a standardized technique, the elbow is flexed to 90 degrees and there is no slack in the ulnar nerve. Extension of the elbow produces a laxity of the ulnar nerve. Conduction determinations with the arm fully extended would result in false values.

CLINICAL USES OF ELECTRONEUROMYOGRAPHY

Electroneuromyography is useful in the following ways:
1. For confirming a clinical diagnosis.
2. For localizing the level of a specific lesion.
3. For distinguishing partial and complete lesions.
4. For distinguishing peripheral nerve anomalies.
5. For intraoperative evaluation of neural lesions.
6. For differentiating primary muscle or nerve pathology.
7. For evaluating malingerers or exaggerators.

Confirming a Clinical Diagnosis

The principal cause of an inability to extend the fingers and thumb at the metacarpophalangeal joint and to dorsiflex the wrist in a radial direction is paralysis of the posterior interosseous nerve. This can be confirmed with electroneuromyography. The extensor digitorum communis would be observed for fibrillations, positive sharp waves, polyphasic potentials, and prolonged conduction time across the elbow — all are confirmatory findings of a nerve entrapment lesion. The motor conduction velocity of this nerve would be delayed in a complete lesion.

Not infrequently, a partial lesion of the same nerve may present only as a drop of one, two, or more digits at the metacarpophalangeal joint. This entity must be distinguished from a rupture of the extensor tendons of these digits at the wrist level. Entrapment of the posterior interosseous nerve and tendon ruptures in rheumatoid arthritis have been reported with increasing frequency in recent years. It is obvious that when the surgeon has confirmation from the electromyographer that there is a nerve lesion at the elbow he can proceed to correct a defect he knows exists instead of attempting to repair a nonexistent tendon rupture.

If electrical studies give normal results, then the lag in extension of the digits at the metacaropohalangeal joint is probably due to pathology of the tendons. Clinically, this can be confirmed by observing finger movement with wrist extension and flexion. With a rupture of the extensor tendon, finger extension will not occur when the wrist is flexed. When a nerve lesion produces the metacarpophalangeal extension lag, the dynamic tenodesis action of the intact extensor tendons will be observed when the wrist is flexed.

Similarly, lack of extension of the thumb alone would suggest a rupture of the extensor pollicis longus tendon at the wrist at Lister's tubercle. However, if pain in the proximal forearm and elbow has preceded the drop in the thumb, and if there is electrical evidence of a denervated extensor pollicis longus, the surgeon has additional clues to plan the appropriate neurosurgical intervention. The accurate diagnosis in this instance would be a partial posterior interosseous nerve paralysis.

The carpal tunnel syndrome cannot always be confirmed by electroneuromyographic procedures. With median nerve compression at the wrist, lack of confirmation has been reported in the past in as many as 25 per cent of cases when motor conduction alone was evaluated. Determinations of electrical sensory disturbance across the wrist improved the correlation.[7] With refined segmental digital-to-palm and palm-to-wrist conduction studies, and with comparison of thumb and long finger sensory conduction values, the correlation has improved to approximately 95 per cent.[2, 3] Therefore, if a patient has a classic carpal tunnel syndrome and yet the EMG does not support it, one must give credence to the clinical diagnosis.

Conduction studies are not always helpful in confirming all compression lesions. It has been reported that median nerve compression at the elbow (lacertus fibrosus, pronator teres, or at the flexor superficialis bridge) is best confirmed by electromyographic abnormalities rather than by disturbances of conduction.[3] The presumptive reason for this questionable lack of correlation is the occurrence of significant numbers of unaffected axons in the nerve, which are believed by some to yield normal conduction velocity results with present techniques.

Localizing the Level of a Specific Lesion

It can be difficult at times to localize the exact level of a lesion. There are numerous variations in the course and nerve fiber contents of the peripheral nerves, and in the innervations of muscles of the forearm and hand. The usual anatomy described in standard medical texts at best is completely present only 40 per cent of the time. Based on clinical examination alone, it is possible not to be absolutely certain of the exact level of the lesion. Conduction delays across a specific segment of the nerve can focus attention on the specific region.

For example, an ulnar nerve lesion at the elbow classically would present with absence of sensation in the ulnar 1½ digits and numbness of the dorsum of the hand and hypothenar eminence of the palm. There would be no clawing of the digits because the flexor digitorum profundus muscles of the fourth and fifth fingers are paralyzed, as are the intrinsic muscles of the hand. However, many variations on both the sensory and the motor sides can be observed in a complete high ulnar nerve lesion — from numbness of only the fifth finger to numbness of the long and ring fingers and even at times a portion of the index finger. Furthermore, clawing can be observed if the median nerve anomalously innervates the flexor digitorum profundus muscles of the fourth and fifth fingers. Similarly, the dorsum of the hand on the ulnar aspect can be supplied by the superficial radial nerve, and sensation clinically would be observed intact on the dorsum of the hand in the region usually supplied by the dorsal cutaneous branch of the ulnar nerve.

Because of these many variations, one must rely on electromyographic and nerve conduction confirmation in many instances.[8]

Electromyography has been helpful in diagnosing unusual cases, such as foramen magnum lesions.[13] The association of intrinsic muscle atrophy with abnormal electromyographic findings consisting of fibrillations and positive sharp waves, as well as normal conduction velocities and high-frequency discharges in the trapezius muscle is suggestive of the high cervical tumor.

With root lesions proximal to the posterior ganglion there are normal evoked sensory responses. Fibrillations, positive sharp waves and complex potentials in the paraspinal musculature are found in lesions proximal to the bifurcation of the posterior division of the spinal nerves. Absence of these findings suggests a more distal lesion.

Distinguishing Partial and Complete Lesions

Electromyography is helpful in distinguishing the degree of physiological completeness of a lesion. The extent of the lesion — whether it is partial or total — can at times be interpreted accurately by electroneuromyographic measures.

If a neural lesion is incomplete, the extent of motor or sensory conduction delay, the latency, the degree of fibrillations or sharp waves, low voltage amplitude, and the type of interference pattern on volitional contraction of muscles are useful in evaluating the extent of injury. The paucity of fibrillation potentials in a neural lesion suggests a neurapractic or first degree lesion.

In a typical posterior interosseous nerve paralysis there is an isolated conduction delay across this nerve. In one typical case the segmental conduction velocity across this nerve was 40 meters per second on the symptomatic side and 60 meters per second on the opposite side. The evoked potentials were small in amplitude and were dispersed in time. No motor unit potentials were found on voluntary muscle contraction. These electrical findings suggested a neurapraxia.

In regard to a partial lesion, one must distinguish an incomplete lesion from a complete one in which a variation exists. Neural variations with anomalous pathways occur frequently. These can be demonstrated by careful electromyographic examination.

Distinguishing Peripheral Nerve Anomalies

The technique for evaluating the presence of a neural anomaly can be demonstrated by describing the EMG recognition of a typical example, the Martin-Gruber communication. In this anomaly, ulnar neural fibers pass from either the anterior interosseous nerve branch or the main median nerve trunk in the proximal forearm and run parallel to the ulnar artery to join the ulnar nerve in the midforearm. Recognition of this rather common anomaly, which occurs in approximately 15 per cent of limbs, can be achieved preoperatively with analysis of the electromyogram.[9] The realization that this cross-pathway exists can at times help clarify an unusual clinical problem.

The Martin-Gruber anomaly can be demonstrated by stimulating the median and ulnar nerves individually above the elbow and at the wrist and recording the response in the abductor digiti quinti or any of the intrinsic muscles that are anomalously innervated. When this variation is present, the amplitude of the evoked potential is greater upon stimulation of the ulnar nerve at the wrist than on stimulation at the elbow.

On occasion, an intrinsic muscle that is usually innervated directly by the ulnar nerve is supplied completely through this Martin-Gruber communication. In this instance, therefore, stimulation of the ulnar nerve of this particular limb above the elbow produces no response. Furthermore, on excitation of the median nerve above the elbow and of the ulnar nerve at the wrist there is an identical response in the specific intrinsic muscle. Stimulation of the median nerve at the wrist produces no response in this anomalously innervated intrinsic muscle.

This method can be utilized for evaluating variant sensory pathways by stimulating the peripheral nerve and recording over the skin segment in question (antidromic method). It can be confirmed also by an ortho-dromic technique. The sensory antidromic method is used more com-monly because the evoked response is larger and easier to evaluate.

A special collision technique electromyography has also proved help-ful in identifying median-to-ulnar nerve crossings in the forearm.[12] The less frequent ulnar-to-median nerve communication can be identified by similar methods.

Dual innervation of muscles, such as the innervation of the first dorsal interosseous, flexor digitorum profundus, lumbricals and other in-trinsic muscles, can be evaluated and clarified by electromyographic analysis.

Intraoperative Evaluation of Neural Lesions

Intraoperative determination of nerve conduction across a partial nerve lesion or a complete neuroma-in-continuity can be evaluated on both gross peripheral nerve and funicular levels.[11, 19] Isolated nerve ac-tion potential recordings across a nerve segment that has been injured can give the operating surgeon valuable information concerning the extent of integrity and the degree of maturation of axons in a damaged neural segment. At a funicular level, intraoperative recordings have also been reported to be of help in managing partial lesions of nerves.[19]

When it is essential for children under the age of 5 years to have electromyography, it may be necessary to conduct the tests under general anesthesia. In children over 5 years cooperation can be elicited, and the need for anesthesia can be avoided through the use of sedatives and by gentleness on the part of the electromyographer. Children's tolerances of pain or multiple needle injections is extremely limited. Obtain only the minimal number of samplings, preferably by surface electrodes; howev-er, where necessary, one or possibly two percutaneous muscle samplings can be obtained.

Differentiating Between Primary Muscle or Nerve Pathology

Electroneuromyography can help differentiate systemic disease processes of either predominantly muscle or predominantly nerve origin. If the process is diffuse, abnormalities in the electromyogram will be found in more than one extremity and frequently in more than one nerve in a particular limb. The neuropathies that may be clinically present with objective findings in one limb may have subclinical manifestations in another. The electromyography may uncover this subclinical aspect of the diffuse disease. Thus, through this technique a systemic diffuse disease process, rather than simply a localized mononeuropathy, can be brought to the attention of the clinician.

A patient with a diffuse disease, such as diabetes, can develop a superimposed localized compression process, as, for example, a carpal tunnel syndrome. The electroneuromyographic evaluation may not be helpful because of the marked conduction delay that exists in the nerve due to the diffuse peripheral neuropathy. Any superimposed delay due to the localized compression lesion may be masked by this slow conduction. In this instance the clinical signs (e.g., pain and numbness of the radial 3½ digits and increased night pain in the hand, requiring the patient to shake the wrist during the night to relieve the increased discomfort) are helpful in recognizing the dual pathology. Some temporary improvement with conservative measures such as splinting of the wrist in a neutral position and use of a diuretic, as well as the presence of other positive confirmatory signs (the Tinel sign localized to the wrist or the positive Phalen sign — increased pain with flexion of the wrist), are of value in diagnosis. If such signs are present in a diabetic, carpal tunnel release may be indicated judiciously, without need for corroborative electromyographic evidence.

The myopathic disorders such as myotonic dystrophy and congenital myotonia are characterized by the classic "dive-bomber" sound. This finding alone helps to localize the disease process to primarily muscle rather than to nerve.

Evaluating Malingerers or Exaggerators

At times the examiner has to evaluate muscle or nerve function in order to confirm or to reject a clinical impression that the neurological complaints given are not bona fide. Conduction studies are objective, and if there is a significant conduction delay or latency across a neural segment these findings must be accepted. However, a patient can voluntarily refrain from contracting a muscle, and therefore, there may be no obliteration of the baseline on the oscilloscope when a muscle is being evaluated. Thus, the normal recruitment may not occur because the patient is voluntarily not contracting the muscle. If the patient has a normal conduction velocity in addition to voluntary oscillographic non-obliteration of the baseline upon requesting the patient to utilize the muscle, these findings would, in conjuction with a bizarre, nonorganic pattern of the clinical examination, suggest that the symptoms are nonorganic in origin.

In conclusion, the electroneuromyographic testings should be considered as only one part in the overall evaluation of the patient with a peripheral nerve problem; they cannot replace clinical examinations. Essentially, they should be utilized to confirm a suspected clinical diagnosis. They make their greatest and indeed sometimes only contribution when they are placed in context with competent serial clinical examinations. Although electroneuromyography is not an end unto itself, it should be included as part of the diagnostic process when evaluating peripheral nerve lesions.

BIBLIOGRAPHY

1. Buchthal, F., and Rosenfalck, A.: Spontaneous Electrical Activity of Human Muscle. Electroenceph. Clin. Neurophysiol., 20:321–336, 1966.
2. Buchthal, F., and Rosenfalck, A.: Sensory Conduction from Digit to Palm and from Palm to Wrist in the Carpal Tunnel Syndrome. J. Neurol. Neurosurg. Psychiat., 34:243–252, 1971.
3. Buchthal, F., Rosenfalck, A., and Trojaborg, W.: Electrophysiological Findings in Entrapment of the Median Nerve at Wrist and Elbow. J. Neurol. Neurosurg. Psychiat., 37:340–360, 1974.
4. Delagi, E. F., and Perotta, A.: Clinical Electromyography of the Hand. Arch. Phys. Med., 57:66–69, 1976.
5. Delagi, E. F., Perotta, A. O., Iazzett, J., and Morrison, D.: Anatomical Guide for the Electromyographer. Springfield, Ill., Charles C Thomas, 1975.
6. Fullerton, P.M., and Gilliatt, R.W.: Axon Reflexes in Human Motor Fibers. J. Neurol. Neurosurg. Psychiat., 28:1–11, 1965.
7. Gilliatt, R.W., and Sears, T.A.: Sensory Nerve Action Potentials in Patients with Peripheral Nerve Lesions. J. Neurol. Neurosurg. Psychiat., 21:109–118, 1958.
8. Gilliatt, R.W., and Thomas, P.K.: Changes in Nerve Conduction with Ulnar Nerve Lesions at the Elbow. J. Neurol. Neurosurg. Psychiat., 23:312–320, 1960.
9. Goodgold, J., and Eberstein, A.: Electrodiagnosis of Neuromuscular Diseases. Baltimore, Williams & Wilkins, 1972.
10. Herbison, G.J., and Staas, W.E.: Electrical Testing: Neuromuscular Physiology and Clinical Application. In Littler, J.W., Cramer, L.M., and Smith, J.W. (Eds.): Symposium on Reconstructive Hand Surgery. St. Louis, Mosby, 1974. pp. 20–51.
11. Kline, D.G., and Hackett, E.R.: Reappraisal of Timing for Exploration of Civilian Peripheral Nerve Injuries. Surgery, 78:54–65, 1975.
12. Kimura, J., Murphy, M.J., and Varda, D.I.: Electrophysiological Study of Anomalous Innervation of Intrinsic Hand Muscles. Arch. Neurol., 33:842–844, 1976.
13. Liveson, J.A., Ransohoff, J., and Goodgold, J.: Electromyographic Studies in a Case of Foramen Magnum Meningioma. J. Neurol. Neurosurg. Psychiat., 36:561–564, 1973.
14. London, G.W.: Normal Ulnar Nerve Conduction Velocity Across the Thoracic Outlet: Comparison of Two Measuring Techniques. J. Neurol. Neurosurg. Psychiat., 38:756–760, 1975.
15. Nakano, K.K., Lundergan, E., and Okihiro, M.M.: Anterior Interosseous Nerve Syndromes: Diagnostic Methods and Alternative Treatments. Arch. Neurol., 34:477–480, 1977.
16. O'Brien, M.D., and Upton, A.R.M.: Anterior Interosseous Nerve Syndrome. J. Neurol. Neurosurg. Psychiat., 35:531–536, 1972.
17. Simpson, J.A.: Fact and Fallacy in Measurement of Conduction Velocity in Motor Nerves. J. Neurol. Neurosurg. Psychiat., 27:381–385, 1964.
18. Trojaborg, W.: Prolonged Conduction Block with Axonal Degeneration. J. Neurol. Neurosurg. Psychiat., 40:50–57, 1977.
19. Williams, H.B., and Terzis, J.K.: Single Fascicular Recordings: An Intraoperative Diagnostic Tool for the Management of Peripheral Nerve Lesions. Plast. Reconstr. Surg., 57:562–569, 1976.

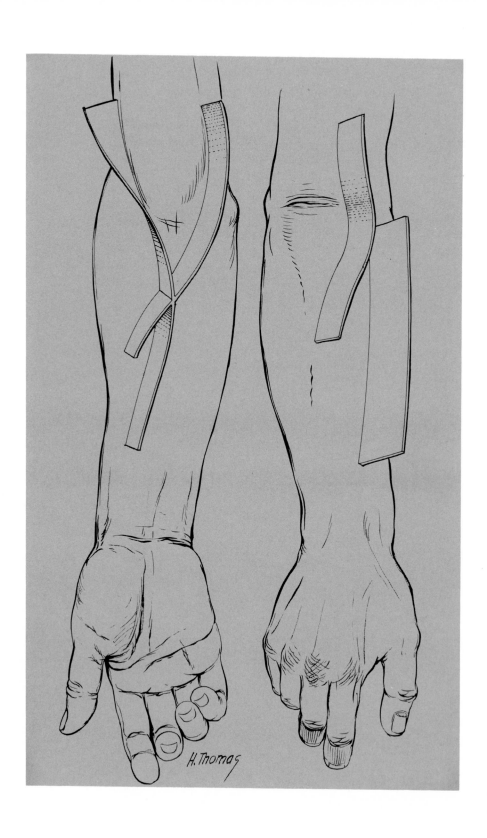

THE INTERNERVOUS PLANES OF THE FOREARM

THE INTERNERVOUS PLANES OF
THE FOREARM

Knowledge of the internervous planes of the forearm can be of immense aid to the upper limb surgeon. These planes represent borders between muscle groups innervated by different major peripheral nerves. The peripheral nerves of the forearm and their branches do not cross these planes. Therefore, familiarity with these planes allows one to move with deftness, confidence, and precision up and down the forearm in order to expose bones, anomalies, pathology, and the appropriate major nerves of the forearm. There are five internervous planes of the forearm.

To illustrate them, we will commence at the subcutaneous border of the ulna (Fig. 12). This first plane separates muscles innervated by the ulnar nerve volarly and the radial nerve dorsally.

The entire ulna can be exposed through this plane without endangering a peripheral nerve or its major branches. Most commonly this approach is utilized in its fullest extent in the treatment of fractures and congenital partial agenesis of the ulna with associated ulnar club hand. Through this means the fibrotic band of the distal ulna can be excised. The incision can be extended proximally and distally through the interosseous plane of the forearm, and the radius can be osteotomized and translocated, creating a one-bone forearm for the congenital defect of the ulna.[3]

This approach is utilized not only for exposure of the entire shaft of the ulna but also for exposure of the radial head and the proximal third of the shaft of the radius.[1]

The second internervous cleavage progressing dorsally is between the anconeus and the extensor carpi ulnaris. Even though both muscles are innervated by the radial nerve, an internervous plane exists between the two. The radial nerve branch to the anconeus passes from the lower arm longitudinally, while the extensor carpi ulnaris is supplied by a branch of the posterior interosseous nerve at the distal border of the superficial head of the supinator, at approximately the junction of the middle and proximal third of the forearm (Fig. 13).

Excision of the radial head is most frequently performed through this second plane. The interval is identified distally and then traced proximally for its clearest definition. After it is developed, the forearm is pronated, bringing the posterior interosseous nerve farther anteriorly,

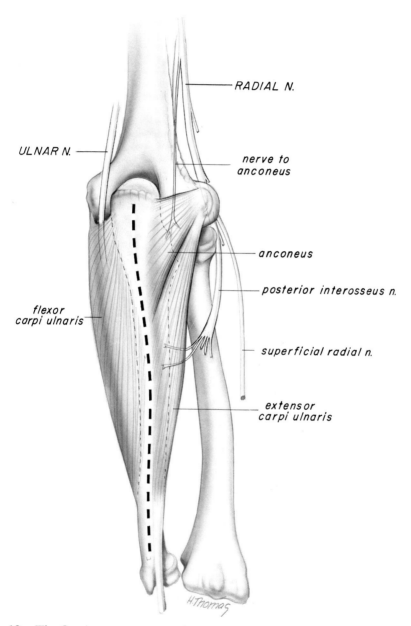

RADIAL N.

ULNAR N.

nerve to
anconeus

anconeus

posterior interosseus n.

flexor
carpi ulnaris

superficial radial n.

extensor
carpi ulnaris

H.Thomas

Figure 12.   The first internervous zone is at the subcutaneous border of the ulna, which separates the ulnar nerve innervated flexor carpi ulnaris and the radial nerve innervated muscles.

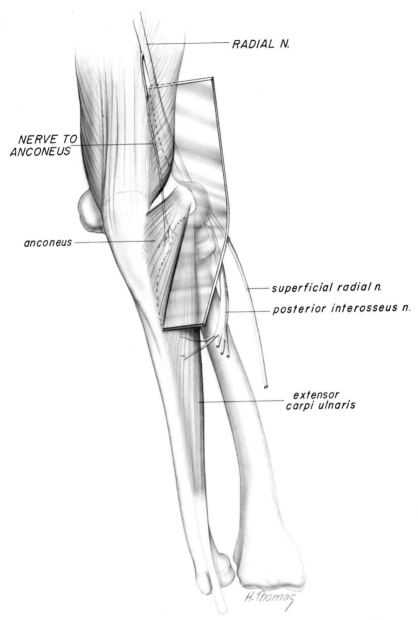

— RADIAL N.

NERVE TO
ANCONEUS

anconeus

superficial radial n.

posterior interosseus n.

extensor
carpi ulnaris

H. Thomas

Figure 13.   The second internervous plane is between the anconeus and the extensor carpi ulnaris. The anconeus is supplied by a branch from the main radial nerve trunk, while the extensor carpi ulnaris is supplied by the posterior interosseous nerve in the forearm.

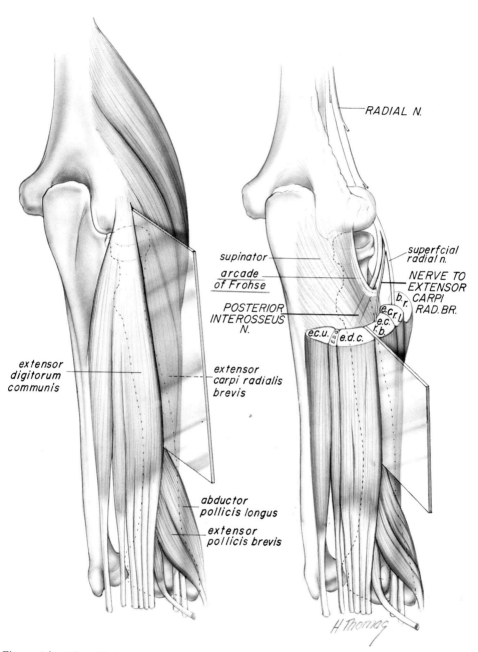

Figure 14. The third internervous plane of the forearm is between the extensor digitorum communis and the extensor carpi radialis brevis. After opening the common raphe completely between these two muscles, the supinator muscle is visualized with the posterior interosseous nerve passing deep to the proximal edge through the arcade of Frohse. The entire course of this nerve can be visualized through this exposure. (e.c.u. = extensor carpi ulnaris; EDQ = extensor digitorum quinti; e.d.c. = extensor digitorum communis; e.c.r.b. = extensor carpi radialis brevis; e.c.r.l. = extensor carpi radialis longus; b.r. = brachioradialis).

away from possible injury. A portion of the supinator adjacent to the ulna is incised longitudinally and then the capsule is incised, thus completing the arthrotomy of the radiocapitular joint.

The third internervous plane, continuing in the same dorsal direction, is between two different branches of the radial nerve. This plane lies between the extensor digitorum communis and the extensor carpi radialis brevis (Fig. 14). The posterior interosseous nerve supplies the extensor digitorum communis after it passes between the heads of the supinator muscle at its distal end. The extensor carpi radialis brevis is supplied by a separate branch, usually from the superficial radial nerve, but the nerve can arise from the region of the bifurcation of the two.

This third internervous plane is first identified distally at the level of the outcropping muscles of the forearm, and is then traced proximally to the level of the lateral epicondyle. In the proximal third of the forearm there is a common aponeurosis between the extensor digitorum communis and the extensor carpi radialis brevis. The muscular fibers of the extensor carpi radialis brevis attaching to this common aponeurosis must be separated in order to identify the deeper plane of the supinator in this proximal region of the forearm.

The posterior interosseous nerve can be identified as it passes through the arcade of Frohse. This approach is also utilized for exposure of the shaft of the radius and for soft tissue tumors adjacent to the radial nerve in the dorsoradial aspect of the soft tissues of the forearm. It is important to identify the posterior interosseous nerve in this approach before proceeding with definitive surgery in this region because of the nerve's vulnerability.

For exposure of the shaft of the radius, the forearm is supinated. The insertion of the supinator is detached and subperiosteal stripping is performed, commencing volar and proceeding dorsally to expose this bone. It must be remembered that the posterior interosseous nerve passes in a dorsoradial direction and that at the level of the biceps tuberosity it can come in direct contact with the dorsoradial aspect of the radius. When clear exposure of this area is necessary, it is wise to identify the posterior interosseous nerve through its course between the two heads of the supinator muscle. The nerve is then retracted, giving safe access to the region (pp. 85–94).

In the distal half of the forearm the outcropping muscles which control extension and abduction of the thumb present themselves (Fig. 14). The internervous plane continues distally along the radial border of the abductor pollicis longus. The extensor carpi radialis longus and brevis tendons pass anterior to the outcropping muscles. To expose the dorsal surface of the midthird of the radius, the extensor carpi radialis tendons are retracted radially and the thumb muscles are brought medially.

In the distal third of the radius the lateral aspect of this bone can be exposed through this plane.

Proceeding farther in the same direction, the volar aspect of the forearm appears where the fourth internervous plane is found. It lies *between the brachioradialis, innervated by a branch of the radial nerve, and flexor-pronator group of muscles innervated by the median nerve (Fig. 15). The pronator teres in the proximal half of the forearm and the

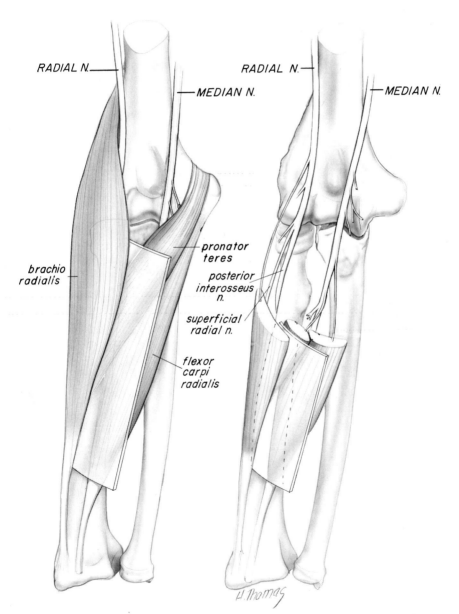

RADIAL N.

MEDIAN N.

RADIAL N.

MEDIAN N.

brachio radialis

pronator teres

posterior interosseus n.

superficial radial n.

flexor carpi radialis

H. Thomas

Figure 15.   The fourth cleavage plane is between the radial nerve innervated brachioradialis and the lateral border of the flexor-pronator group of muscles innervated by the median nerve.

flexor carpi radialis in the distal half are the major muscles innervated by the median nerve and form the medial aspect of this internervous plane.

In developing the proximal third of this region, the superficial radial and the posterior interosseous nerves can be identified. Bicipital bursas, localized hemangiomas, and other soft tissue tumors can be excised by first developing this plane, identifying the vital neural structures, and then excising the tumor; thus, these critical neural structures are left intact.

Exposure of the entire anterior aspect of the radius is achieved through this fourth internervous plane.[2] In the proximal third of the forearm it is the supinator insertion that is stripped radially to expose the proximal third of the forearm. In the middle third, the pronator teres can be elevated medially and the deeper origin of the flexor superficialis can be stripped off the shaft. In the distal end of the radius, the pronator quadratus is elevated to expose the entire length of the radius from an anterior approach. With fractures of the radial head involving the posterior interosseous nerve, the nerve can be identified, released from scar, and retracted safely. The capsule can be opened and the comminuted fragments of the radial head excised through this internervous plane developed in the proximal third of the forearm.

The fifth and final plane, between the median nerve innervated flexor muscles and the ulnar nerve innervated flexor muscles, is identified next. The interval is between the flexor digitorum superficialis muscles (innervated by the median nerve) and the flexor carpi ulnaris (supplied by the ulnar nerve) (Fig. 16). The plane is developed distally and dissected proximally through the entire forearm. The ulnar nerve is identified posterior to the flexor carpi ulnaris on the flexor digitorum profundus muscles. The exposure of the entire course of the ulnar nerve through the forearm is achieved by developing this internervous plane. Soft tissue tumors of the anterior aspect of the forearm on the ulnar side can be visualized through this exposure. Exposure of the ulnar nerve in the forearm is achieved by developing this plane. When anterior translocation of this nerve from behind the elbow is required, as when it is necessary to overcome a gap in the nerve, exposure of the entire forearm is required. A similar interval is utilized when the distal end of the ulna requires visualization anteriorly in the lower third of the forearm. When the ulnar nerve is compressed, as with an anterior locked dislocation of the distal radioulnar joint, such limited exposure of this cleavage plane is valuable. In the lower third of the forearm, the flexor carpi ulnaris and then the ulnar nerve and artery are identified and retracted, exposing the capsule and the dislocated distal radioulnar joint. Using this approach for developing this internervous plane, direct visualization and evaluation of the ulnar nerve are achieved. If supplementary intraoperative electrical testing is necessary, it can be accomplished in this manner,

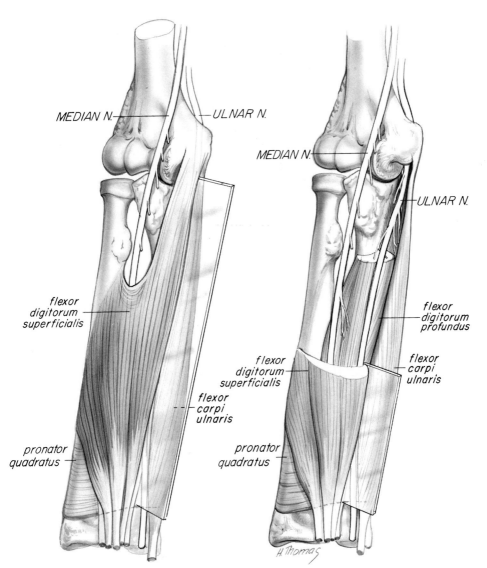

Figure 16.   The fifth internervous plane of the forearm is between the medial border of the flexor digitorum superficialis (supplied by the median nerve) and the adjacent flexor carpi ulnaris, which is innervated by the ulnar nerve.

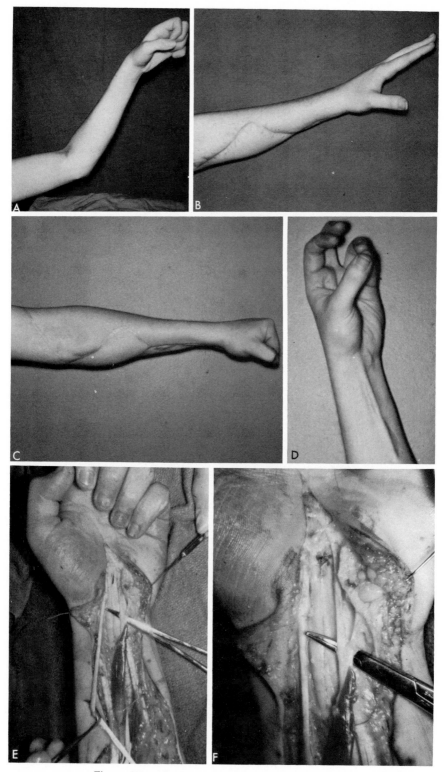

Figure 17.   *Illustration continued on opposite page.*

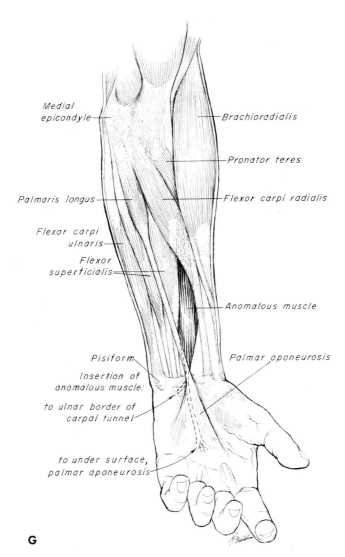

Medial
epicondyle

Brachioradialis

Pronator teres

Palmaris longus

Flexor carpi radialis

Flexor carpi
ulnaris

Flexor
superficialis

Anomalous muscle

Pisiform

Palmar aponeurosis

Insertion of
anomalous muscle:

to ulnar border of
carpal tunnel

to under surface,
palmar aponeurosis

G

Figure 17. *A*, Three weeks following an intra-arterial injection of oral Nembutal the patient had marked restriction of extension of the wrist, fingers, and thumb. He had a Volkmann's ischemic contracture of the forearm musculature. *B*, One year following surgery, marked improvement of extension of the wrist, digits, and thumb is exhibited. *C*, He flexes his fingers well and can oppose his thumb well, *D. E*, An anomalous muscle is seen in the lower third of the forearm. In the carpal tunnel a hemostat is under the tendon of this anomalous muscle. *F*, Close-up view of the carpal tunnel establishes that actually there were two tendons of insertion of this anomalous muscle: one inserted into the ulnar portion of the carpal tunnel; the other passed through the carpal tunnel to attach to the undersurface of the palmar aponeurosis. *G*, Composite drawing of a left forearm demonstrating the anomalous muscle (the palmaris profundus) that was found.

and the surgeon can both clearly evaluate the nerve and excise the distal end of the ulna through the same incision.

Making use of these multiple internervous planes of the forearm in a longitudinal manner readily permits identification of vital structures of the forearm.[4] It allows visualization of multiple neural structures that may require neurolysis. The wide exposure made possible by developing the internervous planes is extremely valuable. Accurate identification of muscle variations which may play a part in deformities such as muscle contractures of Volkmann's ischemia can be clearly visualized. Release of these contracted anomalous structures can yield an excellent postoperative result.

The following case report is a most instructive example of the concept of exposing internervous planes of the forearm in reconstructive surgery. A 23-year-old white male injected the contents of three oral capsules of Nembutal intra-arterially into his left arm. He was initially admitted to a psychiatric hospital for 3 weeks. During that period marked swelling of the arm and forearm was noted. Even though he had been unconscious, at no time had he been lying directly on the arm.

Immediately after the injection the patient recalls that there was burning in his forearm. Gradually his wrist and fingers flexed increasingly despite extension dynamic splints which had been applied to them (Fig. 17A). When I first examined the patient, sensation in the hand was markedly diminished but not totally absent from the areas supplied by the median and ulnar nerves in the hand. There was evidence of marked diminution of thenar and hypothenar motor function and extension of the fingers and wrist. This was observed both clinically and electro-neuromyographically.

Surgery was performed 3 weeks after injury. The procedure was extensive and included release of the median, ulnar, and radial nerves in the forearm. In addition, a flexor-pronator muscle slide procedure in the proximal forearm and distal tendon lengthenings of isolated contracted flexors in the distal forearm were performed (Fig. 17). In the course of the operative procedure, an anomalous muscle, the palmaris profundus, was found to be involved in the ischemic muscle contracture process (Fig. 17E–G). It arose from the deep skeletal plane at the junction of the middle and proximal thirds of the forearm. Its tendinous origin was from the radius and adjacent intermuscular membrane at the level of the takeoff of the anterior interosseous nerve 7 cm. distal to the intercondylar line of the humerus. The muscle extended distally and became tendinous at the level of the distal palmar crease of the wrist. The tendon passed through the carpal tunnel and inserted for the most part on the underside of the palmaris aponeurosis. A separate small insertion was to the ulnar side of the carpal tunnel. This muscle was innervated by a branch of the median nerve.

It should be noted that the major Volkmann's contracture pathology centered on the flexor digitorum profundus and the flexor pollicis longus. In addition, there was a definite infarct of the proximal portion of this anomalous muscle, which arose between the flexor pollicis longus and the flexor profundus adjacent to the anterior interosseous nerve and artery. The wrist could not be fully extended until this anomalous infarcted muscle was detached from the palmar aponeurosis, despite performing proximally a medial flexor muscle release and slide, plus lengthening of the flexor pollicis longus and flexor digitorum profundus tendons distally. It should be noted that the flexor superficialis muscles did not contribute to the flexion deformities at either the wrist or the finger level. Pathologically, the excised anomalous muscle was reported to show the microscopic changes seen in Volkmann's contracture. The patient had external neurolysis, with release and translocation (1) of the ulnar nerve from behind the medial epicondyle, (2) the median nerve through the area of the lacertus fibrosus, pronator teres, and the flexor superficialis arch and (3) the posterior interosseous branch of the radial nerve through the arcade of Frohse at the proximal level of the supinator.

By utilizing the concept of wide operative exposures of internervous planes of the forearm accomplishing successfully multiple neurolyses, muscle slide, tendon lengthenings, and identification of anomalous muscles in the deformed limb, corrective surgery can be performed accurately, producing excellent functional results (Fig. 17B–D).

BIBLIOGRAPHY

1. Boyd, H.B.: Surgical Exposure of the Ulna and Proximal Third of the Radius Through One Incision. Surg. Gynecol. Obstet., 71:86–88, 1940.
2. Henry, A.K.: Extensile Exposure. 2nd Ed. Baltimore, Williams & Wilkins, 1970, pp. 100–106.
3. Spinner, M., Freundlich, B.D., and Abeles, E.D.: Management of Moderate Longitudinal Arrest of Development of the Ulna. Clin. Orthop., 69:199–202, 1970.
4. Spinner, M.: Importance of Muscle Variations as a Factor in the Deformity of Volkmann's Contracture. Bull. Hosp. Joint Dis., 34:48–54, 1973.

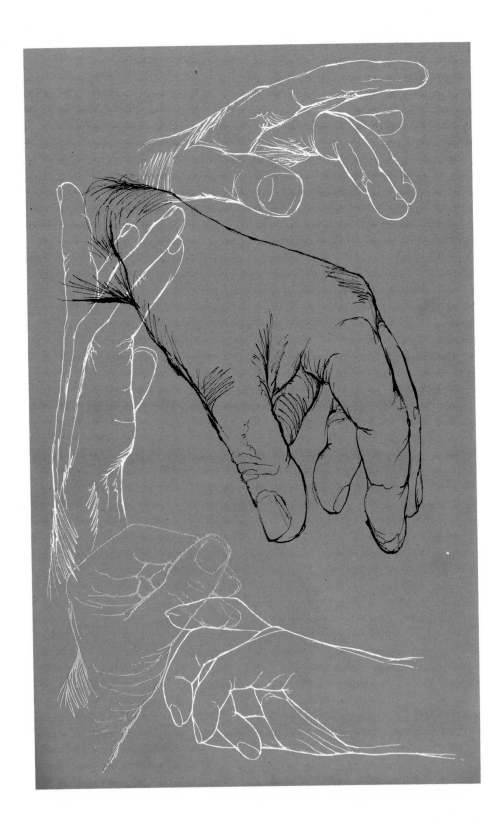

Section VIII

THE RADIAL NERVE

THE RADIAL NERVE

ANATOMY

The radial nerve arises from the posterior cord of the brachial plexus. It receives neural fibers from the cervical roots of C5 to C8. The radial nerve in the arm winds posterior to the humerus, with the deep brachial artery just distal to the musculospiral groove. The nerve comes anterior to the distal arm 10 cm. proximal to the lateral epicondyle after piercing the lateral intermuscular septum. In the arm it supplies the three heads of the triceps and the anconeous. In addition, sensory nerves—the posterior cutaneous nerve of the arm and forearm—are supplied.

In the distal third of the arm proximal to the elbow epicondylar line, the radial nerve innervates the brachioradialis and the extensor carpi radialis longus. On occasion it furnishes a branch to the radial portion of the brachialis muscle, whose major and most constant supply is the musculocutaneous nerve. In the majority of limbs (58 per cent) the motor innervation to the extensor carpi radialis brevis arises from the sensory division of the radial nerve in the forearm, the superficial radial nerve[71] (Fig. 18B).

At the elbow the radial nerve bifurcates into its sensory and motor components, usually at the level of the radiocapitellar joint, but in some cases 2 to 5 cm. proximal or distal to this joint.[9, 32] The posterior interosseous nerve enters and passes between the two heads of the supinator muscle (Fig. 19A). It continues dorsolaterally around the neck of the radius and innervates the supinator while coursing through it. The extensor carpi radialis brevis usually receives its innervation at the level of the radial head or distal to it.

About 8 cm. below the elbow joint, as the radial nerve emerges from the supinator, it divides into multiple branches which resemble a cauda equina (Fig. 19B). As noted by personal observation and dissection, the basic pattern of division consists of two major components — those supplying the superficial layer of muscles (the extensor digitorum communis, the extensor digiti quinti, and the extensor carpi ulnaris) and those deeper to the outcropping muscles of the skeletal plane (the abductor pollicis longus, the extensor pollicis longus and brevis, and the extensor indicis proprius).

At the wrist the posterior interosseous nerve gives off terminal sensory branches to the ligaments of the radiocarpal, intercarpal, and

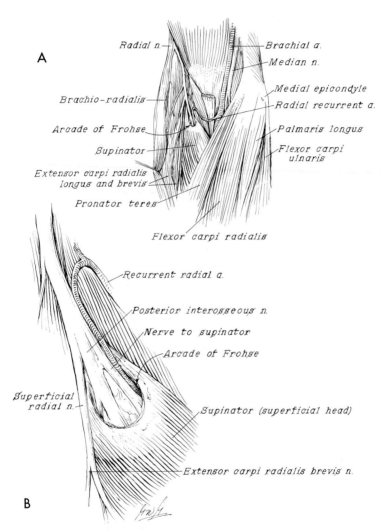

Figure 18.   *A*, Composite drawing of dissections of the forearm at the level of the elbow. *B*, Enlarged view of posterior interosseous nerve and its relationship to the supinator muscle. The arcade of Frohse is readily seen. The motor supply to the extensor carpi radialis brevis arises most frequently from the superficial radial nerve.

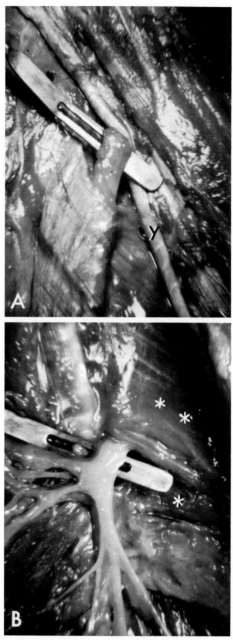

Figure 19.   *A*, Right arm anatomical specimen. The posterior interosseous nerve under the eye of the probe is seen to pass deep to the superficial head of the supinator muscle. The tendinous origin of the extensor carpi radialis brevis (y) is in close proximity to the posterior interosseous nerve. *B*, The posterior interosseous nerve at the lower end of the superficial head of the supinator (**) terminates into multiple branches resembling a cauda equina. The lateral longitudinally oriented branches innervate the abductor pollicis longus, extensor pollicis brevis, extensor pollicis longus and extensor indicis proprius while the horizontally oriented medial branches supply the extensor digitorum communis, extensor digiti quinti and extensor carpi ulnaris. The deep head of the supinator muscle (*) extends more distally than the superficial head. At the lower border of the deep head of the supinator muscle the posterior interosseous vessels first come in proximity to the posterior interosseous nerve.

carpometacarpal joints (Fig. 20). The nerve branches to the extensor digitorum communis muscle are in part recurrent as they enter the middle third of this muscle. The proximal third of the extensor digitorum communis is innervated by this recurrent nerve component (Figs. 29*A* and 41*E*).

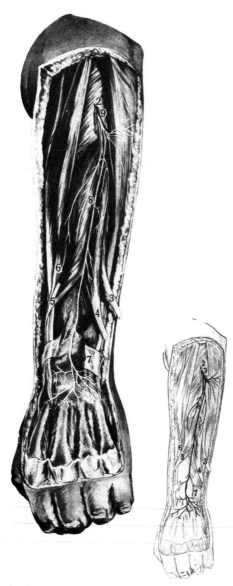

Figure 20. The posterior interosseous nerve gives off terminal sensory branches to the ligaments of the radiocarpal, intercarpal, and carpometacarpal joints distal to the extensor retinaculum (7). (From V. N. Shevkunenko: Atlas of the Peripheral Nervous and Venous System. Moscow, Medgiz, 1949.) These terminal sensory branches have clinical significance. They are vulnerable to injury with neuroma formation in as benign a procedure as ganglion removal on the dorsal or dorsoradial aspect of the wrist.

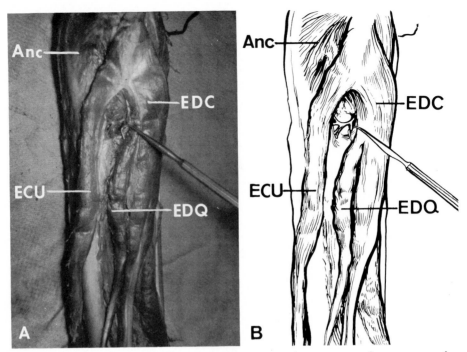

Figure 21.   Anatomical dissection of a right forearm demonstrates the nerve supply to the extensor carpi ulnaris and the extensor digiti quinti. The hook is about the nerve to the extensor digiti quinti. These branches are about 8 cm. distal to the lateral epicondyle.

The extensor carpi ulnaris is supplied by one to three terminal branches of the posterior interosseous nerve which pass horizontally in a medial direction (Fig. 21). They arise from the posterior interosseous nerve on a level just distal to the most distal portion of the insertion of the anconeus. The branches run proximally and distally within the muscle. The extensor digiti quinti is supplied by a branch of the posterior interosseous nerve just radial to the supply to the extensor carpi ulnaris. These motor branches are vulnerable to injury if the intervals between the extensor carpi ulnaris and the extensor digiti quinti, or between the extensor digiti quinti and the extensor digitorum communis in the midforearm, are opened. The safe internervous planes in this area are between the anconeus and the extensor carpi ulnaris and between the extensor digitorum communis and the extensor carpi radialis brevis (see Figs. 13 and 14).

Two major branches of the posterior interosseous nerve supply the outcropping muscles of the skeletal plane. At the level of the distal border of the superficial head of the supinator, a lateral and medial branch pass distally. These arise from the radial aspect of the posterior interosseous nerve. The lateral, longitudinally oriented branch supplies the abductor pollicis longus and extensor pollicis brevis. The other branch frequently innervates both the extensor pollicis longus and the extensor indicis proprius. There can be a separate branch from the posterior interosseous nerve to the extensor indicis proprius (Fig. 19B).

The main trunk of the radial nerve which courses to its divisions at the elbow supplies sympathetic fibers to the radial artery proximally. In the forearm the radial artery is supplied segmentally in the middle and distal sections by sympathetic nerve fibers from the superficial radial nerve.[39]

SIGNIFICANT ANATOMICAL VARIATIONS AND CLINICAL APPLICATIONS

Bare area of the proximal radius.
Arcade of Frohse.
Isolated spontaneous paralysis of the posterior interosseous nerve.
Partial posterior interosseous nerve paralysis.
Tardy posterior interosseous nerve palsy.
Resistant tennis elbow.
Variations of the posterior interosseous nerve and superficial radial nerve.
Variations of the muscles of the radial aspect of the elbow.
Froment-Rauber nerve.

The Bare Area of the Proximal Radius

The bare area[18] of the radius lies posterior to the bicipital tuberosity (Fig. 22A). In 25 per cent of dissected adult upper limbs, a bare area 3 × 3/4 cm. has been noted. The bare area occurs when the insertion of the deep head of the supinator is not in contact throughout its extent with the insertion of the superficial head (Fig. 22C and D).

A visible or palpable groove in the radius, posterior to the bicipital tuberosity, may be found; it is an osseous manifestation of this type of insertion of the two heads of the supinator.

Fractures of the proximal radius that require open reduction because of poor fracture contact can be complicated by a posterior interosseous nerve paralysis. In 25 per cent of adult limbs the posterior interosseous nerve lies directly on the periosteum in this region, in the dorsal aspect of the radius opposite the level of the bicipital tuberosity (Fig. 22A and B). If a plate is utilized in fixation of the fracture, and its proximal screw hole is opposite the bicipital tuberosity (Fig. 23), then it is possible, unless particular care is taken, for the nerve to become trapped under the plate.   *Text continued on page 89*

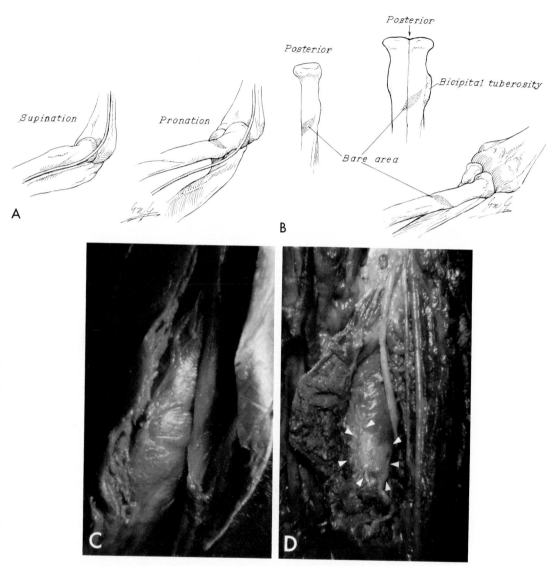

Figure 22.   *A*, In supination when the bare area of the proximal radius is present, the posterior interosseous nerve comes to lie against the periosteum of the radius. *B*, Details of the bare area are noted. *C*, Left forearm specimen. The superficial head of the supinator has been incised completely. The posterior interosseous nerve is found to lie directly on the deep head of the supinator. This occurs in the majority of limbs. *D*, Another left arm specimen demonstrating the bare area which is present when the deep head of the supinator fails to insert completely on the same line of the radius as the superficial head. This specimen is in pronation to demonstrate the details of the bare area.

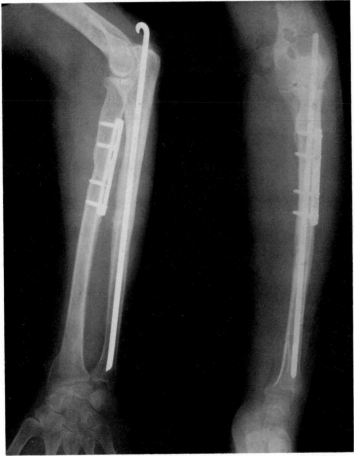

Figure 23.   Healed fracture of both bones of the left forearm. The most proximal screw is at the level of the bicipital tuberosity. It is at this level that the posterior interosseous nerve can be caught under the plate.

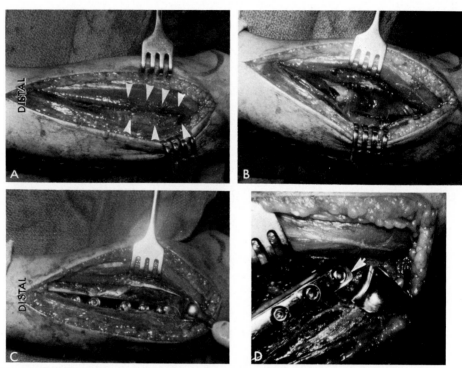

Figure 24.   Fracture of left radius. *A*, The interval between the extensor carpi radialis brevis and the extensor communis digitorum is identified distally and traced proximally to open its raphe accurately. *B*, These superficial muscles are retracted. The fracture of the radius is seen. The supinator muscle is noted about the proximal radius. *C*, After the insertion of the supinator on the radius is detached, the fracture is reduced and plated. *D*, It is under the proximal end of the plate that the posterior interosseous nerve can be caught.

The best treatment for this complication is to avoid its occurrence. Knowing that the nerve can lie against the proximal radius in this region is imperative. If a plate is to be placed on the dorsal surface up to this level, then one must either expose the posterior interosseous nerve or make certain that there is no soft tissue under the uppermost portion of the plate (Fig. 24). If, after plating, a complete posterior interosseous nerve paralysis is observed and if the nerve had not been exposed, then early exploration of the nerve within a day or two is indicated. I have explored several patients with complete posterior interosseous nerve paralysis caused by a radial shaft plate (Fig. 25A–I). Recovery of neural function occurred in such lesions as late as four months after the initial surgery. I have seen posterior interosseous nerve paralysis produced by traction alone, even when the bone plate did not go to the bicipital tuberosity level, owing to excessive traction on the nerve during the surgical procedure. If clinical or electrical function does not return within 3 months after fixation, neurolysis should be performed. Function of the muscles innervated by the posterior interosseous nerve recover following an axonotmetic pattern.

The Arcade of Frohse

As a result of dissections of the radial nerve done on 50 adult arms in the region of the elbow and proximal forearm, a composite illustration of the region has been prepared (Fig. 18A). This drawing demonstrates the radial nerve bifurcating just proximal to the elbow joint and the posterior interosseous nerve entering the supinator through an inverted arch. This arch was described in 1908 by the German anatomist Frohse[22] and is called the arcade of Frohse. The radial recurrent artery crosses this region. In the lower drawing a close view of the entrance of the posterior interosseous nerve into the supinator is demonstrated (Fig. 18B).

In 30 per cent of the adult specimens a fibrous arch was found through which the nerve entered the supinator. This arcade is formed by the tendinous thickened edge of the proximal border of the superficial head of the supinator.

The arcade arises in a semicircular manner from the tip of the lateral epicondyle; its fibers arch downward 1 cm. and then attach to the medial aspect of the lateral epicondyle just lateral to the articular surface of the capitellum. The posterior interosseous nerve passes under the edge of this fibrous arch. The dissected adult specimens revealed considerable variation in the thickness of the fibrous arch and the size of the opening for the passage of the nerve (Figs. 26 and 27).

Text continued on page 94

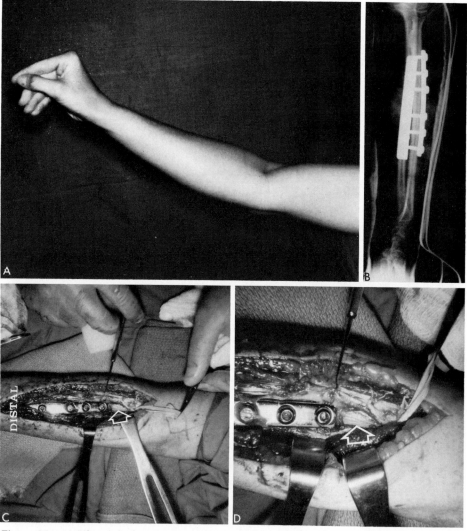

Figure 25.   *A*, The right hand of a patient with a posterior interosseous nerve paralysis. She could not extend her fingers at the metacarpophalangeal joint and had a lag in extension of her thumb. *B*, Roentgenogram revealed that she had had an open reduction of a fracture of both forearms with compression screw-plate fixation. Note the level of the proximal end of the plate to the bicipital tuberosity. *C*, At surgery the posterior interosseous nerve (arrow) has been identified at the arcade of Frohse and traced to the plate. *D*, Closeup view reveals the multifunicular posterior interosseous nerve (arrow)

Illustration continued on opposite page

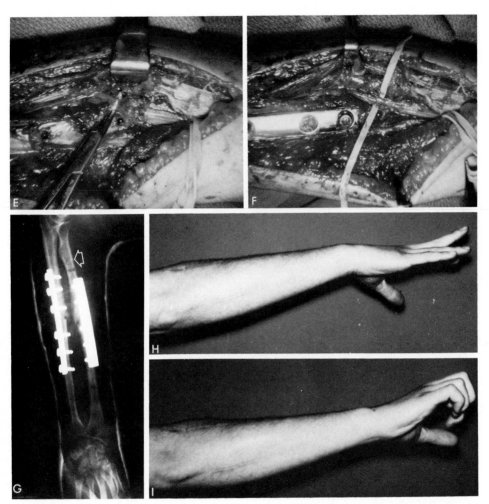

passing directly under the most proximal portion of the plate. *E*, The plate has been removed. Under the hemostat. The markedly compressed posterior interosseous nerve has been identified. The most proximal screw hole is extremely close to the compressed nerve. *F*, An external neurolysis was performed initially and the epineurium over the compressed area was removed, utilizing the operating microscope. A shorter plate (5 hole) was placed, since the fracture fixation was only one month old. *G*, This roentgenogram reveals the level of the most proximal screw hole in the radius and the region just proximal to it (arrow) where the compression of the posterior interosseous nerve had occurred. *H* and *I*, Three months after the neurolysis and replating there is return of function of the posterior interosseous nerve, as indicated by the patient's ability to extend the metacarpophalangeal joints with the fingers extended and with the fingers flexed at the proximal and distal interphalangeal joints.

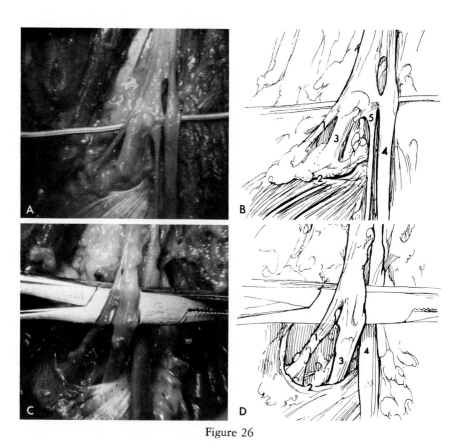

Figure 26

Figures 26 and 27.   Dissected left arm specimens which demonstrate the variations of thickness of the fibrous arch and the size of the opening for passage of the posterior interosseous nerve. 1, A nerve to the supinator muscle; 2, the arcade of Frohse; 3, the posterior interosseous nerve; 4, the superficial radial nerve; and 5, the nerve to the extensor carpi radialis brevis.

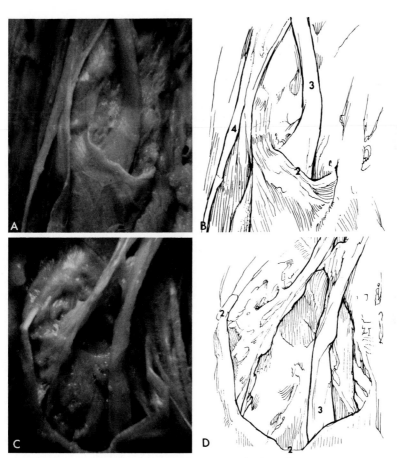

Figure 27.   *See facing page for legend.*

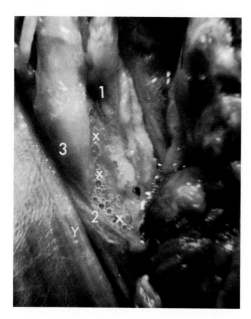

Figure 28. Right arm specimen. In several specimens in full pronation of the forearm the sharp tendinous edge of the origin of the extensor carpi radialis brevis muscle (Y) increased the compression of the posterior interosseous nerve (3). 2, Arcade of Frohse; 1, nerve to the supinator muscle; and x, bubbles of fat produced by the increased compression in full pronation of the forearm.

In addition to its origin along the lateral aspect of the lateral epicondyle, the superficial head of the supinator arises along the radial (lesser sigmoid) notch of the ulna. In 70 per cent of the specimens, the medial half of the arcade was membranous.[78] Paturet[62] noted that on occasion this arcade was a very small "bouton" or button type opening for passage of the nerve.

The extensor carpi radialis brevis muscle frequently has a sharp tendinous medial edge proximally after arising from the lateral epicondyle. In several specimens studied, when the forearm was in full pronation, there was increased pressure and narrowing of the region for the passage of the posterior interosseous nerve (Fig. 28).

In the dissected limbs of ten full-term newborns it was not possible to demonstrate a sharp tendinous arcade of Frohse in any of the specimens. The most proximal part of the superficial head of the supinator was always muscular (Fig. 29).

Isolated Spontaneous Paralysis of the Posterior Interosseous Nerve

Idiopathic or spontaneous paralysis of the posterior interosseous nerve has been described during the last century as "paralysis in the absence of trauma," "non-traumatic progressive paralysis of the posterior interosseous nerve," and "posterior interosseous neuritis." It is my opinion that this lesion most frequently is an entrapment of the posterior interosseous nerve in the proximal forearm as it enters the supinator

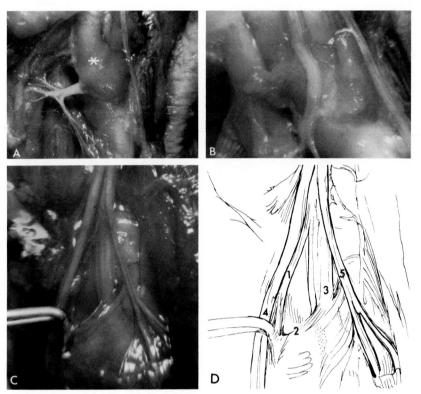

Figure 29.   Right arm: full-term fetal dissection *(A)*. The posterior interosseous nerve is seen as it penetrates the supinator muscle (*). The nerve branches to the extensor digitorum communis muscle are in part recurrent as they enter the middle third of this muscle. The proximal third is innervated by this recurrent component. *B*, The superficial head of the supinator has been cut. The posterior interosseous nerve is seen in continuity. *C* and *D*, There was no tendinous arcade of Frohse (2) noted in the full-term newborn specimens dissected. The posterior interosseous nerve (3) is seen passing deep to the muscular portion of the superficial head of the supinator. The superficial radial nerve (4) and the nerve to the extensor carpi radialis brevis (5) pass superficial to the supinator muscle. 1, A nerve to the supinator muscle.

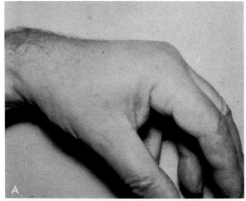
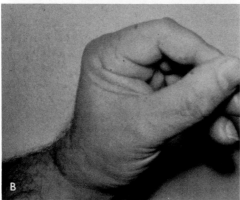

Figure 30. Posterior interosseous nerve paralysis, left hand. Note the ability to fully extend the wrist (B). The fingers do not extend beyond 45 degrees at the metacarpophalangeal joints of the fingers. The thumb cannot be extended to the plane of the metacarpals (A).

muscle (Figs. 18 and 34). On extremely rare occasions the entrapment can occur within the supinator[15] or at its distal end (Fig. 37).

TYPES OF CLINICAL PRESENTATIONS OF POSTERIOR INTEROSSEOUS NERVE PARALYSIS.   The clinical picture has two patterns. The first, from the onset, is that of full-blown, complete paralysis of all the muscles innervated by the posterior interosseous nerve — the extensor digitorum communis, extensor indicis proprius, extensor digiti quinti, extensor carpi ulnaris, abductor pollicis longus, extensor pollicis longus, and extensor pollicis brevis (Fig. 30). The second type commences with paralysis of one or several of the muscles innervated by the posterior interosseous nerve and, if untreated, most frequently progresses to a complete paralysis. When the ring and little fingers are initially involved the hand so affected has been described as a "pseudoulnar claw" (Fig. 31).

Throughout this century there have been isolated reports of spontaneous (idiopathic) complete paralysis of the posterior interosseous nerve.[10, 15, 16, 25, 27, 28, 31, 38, 58, 60, 61, 75, 78, 91, 93] Woltman and Learmonth,[43] Otenasek,[61] and Mulholland[58] have reported such paralysis in cases they explored some 3 to 10 years after onset of paralysis, finding a fibroma or a pseudo-neuroma of the posterior interosseous nerve. As early as 1908,

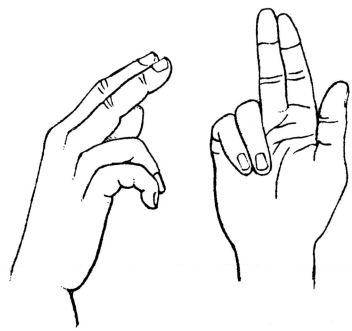

Figure 31.   Note the attitude of the pseudoulnar claw hand observed in a partial posterior interosseous nerve paralysis. There is no hyperextension of the metacarpophalangeal joints of the ring and little fingers, which is usually seen with a low ulnar nerve
lesion. Here, there is lack of full extension of the metacarpophalangeal joints of these
two digits. (Adapted from Marie, P., Meige, H., and Patrikios: Paralysie Radiale Dissociée
Simulant une Griffe Cubitale. Rev. Neurol., *31*:123–124, 1917.)

the German anatomist Frohse[22, 33] described an inverted arch for passage
of the posterior interosseous nerve. At times, this opening could be
extremely narrowed. In 1964 and 1966 Capener[12, 13] likened the sharp
aponeurotic proximal edge of the supinator to the transverse carpal
ligament at the wrist, which is the restraining structure in the carpal
tunnel syndrome. Sharrard, in 1966,[73] noted a fibrous band over the
posterior interosseous nerve in the cases he explored because of persistent localized paralysis of this nerve.

The cases of complete paralysis that were explored 3 to 10 years
after onset failed to respond to neurolysis, probably because of the length
of time of the dysfunction. The pathological findings are compatible with
those found in nerves after prolonged compression.

PATTERNS OF DYSFUNCTION IN COMPLETE POSTERIOR INTEROSSEOUS
NERVE PARALYSIS.   The attitude of the hand afflicted with complete
posterior interosseous nerve paralysis is typical. The wrist dorsiflexes
usually in a radial deviation which can be brought actively to neutral, but
not ulnarly. The fingers can extend at the two distal joints but they
cannot be extended the last 45 degrees (or more) at the metacarpopha-

langeal joint (Figs. 25*A* and 30). The thumb cannot extend in the plane of the metacarpals because of the paralysis of the extensor pollicis longus and brevis muscles. In its position anterior to the plane of the metacarpals, the distal phalanx of the thumb can extend, but not as strongly as usual. This movement is achieved through the function of the intrinsic muscles innervated by the median and ulnar nerves.

Partial Posterior Interosseous Nerve Paralysis

A group of cases were reported by several French neurologists, Marie, Meige, and Patrikios,[50] Roussy and Branche,[70] and Jumentié,[35] between 1917–1921, in which they described a "false ulnar claw hand" due to a "dissociated" lesion of this major motor branch of the radial nerve. These writers described just one type of clinical presentation seen with incomplete paralysis of this nerve. In their cases the fourth and fifth digits were involved. Other single digits, combinations of digits, or the thumb can initially have a lag in extension at the metacarpophalangeal joint, which is a presenting manifestation of partial posterior interosseous nerve paralysis.[19, 25, 27, 31, 58, 61]

PATTERNS OF DYSFUNCTION OF PARTIAL POSTERIOR INTEROSSEOUS NERVE PARALYSIS.   At first glance, the resting attitude of a pseudoulnar claw hand is falsely suggestive of an ulnar nerve paralysis because of the flexion attitude of the ring and little fingers at both the metacarpophalangeal and interphalangeal joints (Fig. 31). However, on further inspection, the lack of a true clawed digit with the usual hyperextension of the metacarpophalangeal joint is noted. The diagnosis of partial posterior interosseous nerve paralysis is confirmed when it is noted that all the ulnar nerve-innervated intrinsic muscles are functioning. Only the extrinsic digital extensor muscles to the ring and little fingers innervated by the posterior interosseous nerve are paralyzed.

The above disorder should not be confused with inability to extend the fifth, fourth, and perhaps the third digit at the metacarpophalangeal joint, which is not uncommonly seen in rheumatoid disease as part of the Vaughan-Jackson syndrome (Fig. 32).[86] A history of multiple joint pain and swelling, derangement of the distal radioulnar joint and roentgenographic changes all help to clarify the pathological condition. It should be remembered that the earlier isolated case reports in the literature of bona fide posterior interosseous nerve paralysis initially described weakness in the fourth and fifth digits before the full-blown paralysis presents itself. Therefore, one should not be surprised that with a partial posterior interosseous paralysis there is initially paresis of these digits.

Other reported cases presented at the onset with weakness of the thumb (Otenasek[61] and Grigoresco et al.[27]), index finger (Mulholland[58]), ring finger (Goldman et al.[25]), and third, fourth, and fifth fingers (Hob-

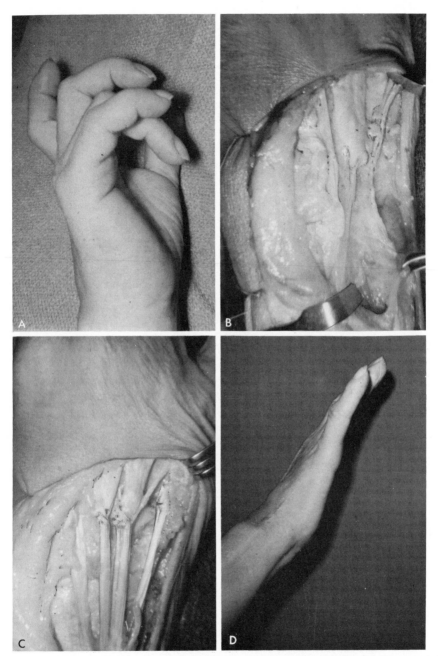

Figure 32. Vaughan–Jackson syndrome. *A,* The right hand is unable to fully extend the long, ring and little fingers at the metacarpophalangeal joints. The patient has long-standing rheumatoid arthritis. *B,* Demonstrates the Vaughan–Jackson lesion. There is direct communication of the distal radioulnar joint with the compartment for the extensor digiti quinti. The communication is seen at the end of the retractor. *C,* The extensor indicis proprius has been transferred to extend the little finger. The ruptured portions of the common extensors were transferred to the adjacent functioning common extensors. *D,* End result demonstrates full extension of the involved digits. The patient could flex fully 3 months after surgery.

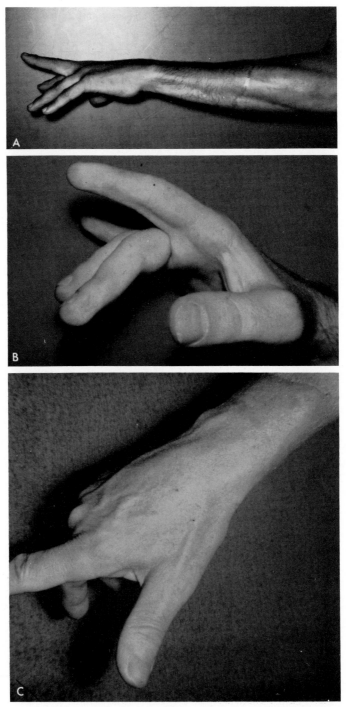

Figure 33.   *A,* Laceration of the middle third of the forearm, which produced a combination of tendon and partial posterior interosseous nerve injury. Only the long finger
can be extended. The index and little fingers suffered denervation of the extensor indicis proprius and extensor digiti quinti, in addition to laceration of part of the common
Legend continued on opposite page

house and Heald,[31] Dharapak and Nimberg,[19] and Nielsen[60]), and then followed gradually with paralysis of extension of some or all of the remaining digits at the metacarpophalangeal level. At the onset of the paralysis, the syndrome of posterior interosseous nerve dysfunction may present with partial paralysis or paresis of one or more of the digits rather than all. Elbow pain at the onset is frequently associated with this entrapment lesion.

If the extensor pollicis longus is the first muscle involved in the partial neural lesion, an incorrect diagnosis of rupture of the extensor pollicis longus tendon may be considered. Furthermore, if an extensor indicis proprius transfer is performed to gain extension of the thumb, a subsequent progression of the paralysis to adjacent digits, with loss of the last 45 degrees of extension of the digits and recurrent loss of extension of the thumb, will be difficult to explain to the patient. Thus, this entrapment lesion at the supinator level due to a fibrotic band or a space-occupying lesion must be considered in differential diagnosis of the more common problem of rupture of the extensor pollicis longus tendon. Electromyographic studies may be necessary when any doubt arises, especially when the inability to extend the thumb is not associated with prior wrist fracture, wrist sprain, or swelling. There need not be pain referred to the proximal forearm with a lesion of this nerve. Only half of the cases had pain in the proximal forearm as a harbinger of the forthcoming paralysis.

If the motor branch to the extensor communis is denervated, drop would occur in the long and ring fingers, with extension of the index and fifth fingers only. The thumb would extend fully at both the metacarpophalangeal and interphalangeal joints. The same type of hand attitude is seen in congenital absence of the common extensor muscles (Fig. 33B) and in lacerations of the extensor surface of the distal forearm in which all the common extensor tendons are injured, with only the extensor indicis proprius and the extensor digiti quinti muscles capable of functioning.

Figure 33   *Continued*

extensor group. The three outcropping muscles of the thumb—the extensor pollicis longus and brevis and the abductor pollicis longus—are deinnervated. The extensor carpi ulnaris is seen functioning. B, The inability to extend the two middle fingers fully can be seen in congenital absence of the extensor digiti communis muscle, in laceration of all the common extensor tendons leaving extension of the index and fifth fingers to their proprius tendons, or in denervation of the extensor digitorum communis muscle. C, Thumb and index finger extend fully. The common extensor tendons are lacerated, as is the extensor digiti quinti. The thumb and the index finger are extended by the extensor pollicis longus and brevis and the extensor indicis proprius respectively.

At times lacerations of the proximal one third of the forearm can produce a combination of both muscle-tendon laceration and denervation of the posterior interosseous nerve or its branches. The pattern of dysfunction of the hand can vary significantly from just one digit not extending fully to all the digits not extending at the metacarpophalangeal joint, with or without involvement of extension of the thumb (Fig. 33A and C). In all of these instances, sensation of the dorsum of the thumb would be maintained because the superficial radial nerve is usually spared.

As has been noted, the extensor carpi radialis longus and brevis muscles will be functioning in a posterior interosseous nerve syndrome, and dorsiflexion of the wrist will be maintained. On the extremely rare occasion when all extensors of the wrist are supplied by the posterior interosseous nerve, a lesion of the nerve would be manifested not only by the presence of dropped fingers but also by dropped wrist. This infrequent type of innervation would have to be considered, and has been reported in Otenasek's case of isolated posterior interosseous nerve palsy, in which a fibroma of this nerve was characterized by dropped fingers and wrist.[61] The differential diagnosis with high radial nerve paralysis, which is much more frequent, must be considered. A high radial nerve lesion is characterized clinically in the forearm and hand by inability to extend the wrist and fingers and by absence of sensation in the autonomous skin area of the dorsoradial aspect of the hand. The presence of a normal radial nerve sensory zone in the hand and a functioning brachioradialis muscle should help to localize the lesion to the posterior interosseous nerve rather than the main radial nerve trunk.

Sunderland,[83, 84] in his study of simple compression injuries of the main radial nerve, noted that the brachioradialis muscle was more prone to severe impairment than other muscles. In contradistinction I have never seen, nor has there been reported, an absence of function of this muscle in a posterior interosseous nerve paralysis.

SYSTEMIC DISEASE AS A CAUSE OF POSTERIOR INTEROSSEOUS NERVE PARALYSIS.   There are isolated paralyses of the posterior interosseous nerve which can occur as a result of systemic disease. These must be considered in differential diagnosis. One systemic disease that may cause an isolated paralysis is *periarteritis nodosa* and it is usually transient. The presence of disease in another organ system should alert the examiner to suspect this disease process.

Diabetes may be either a cause or an additive factor. It should be considered in a patient with a compression syndrome at the elbow, for he may have diabetes as well. The diabetes may be a predisposing factor or just be concomitant to the compression. Electromyographic or clinical evidence of neuropathic involvement in the other extremities in a diabetic would strengthen the diagnosis of diabetes as the cause for the isolated paralysis.

Lead poisoning typically involves the entire radial nerve with a wrist drop or finger drop without sensory abnormalities or peripheral nerve tenderness. In descriptions of lead poisoning by Duchenne[20] there is a note of isolated paralysis of the abductor or the extensor of the thumb, so that partial paralysis of the posterior interosseous nerve may be a manifestation of lead poisoning. Woltman and Kernohan[92] have noted that the paralysis of this heavy metal intoxication usually begins with an inability to extend the long and ring fingers at the metacarpophalangeal joint. Later, there is inability to extend the index and little fingers at this joint level. Subsequently the thumb extensors become involved. In a full-blown lesion, wrist extensor, thenar, and interosseous muscles may be involved. Urinary lead and protoporphyrin (Type III) studies, confirmatory findings of hematological abnormalities consistent with lead intoxication, gum changes, and a history of pica ingestion help to differentiate the condition from a localized entrapment phenomenon and identify it as a manifestation of heavy metal toxicity.

Heavy metal intoxication due to arsenic, thallium, or antimony usually produces polyneuropathic involvement. However, wrist drop has been reported in association with arsenicals.[53]

In the era when *antisera* were utilized in the treatment of diphtheria and scarlet fever, radial nerve and isolated posterior interosseous nerve palsy was observed.

Herpes zoster, sarcoid, and leprosy, although associated with isolated peripheral neuropathies, have not as yet been documented as involving the posterior interosseous nerve.

Hysterical or volitional paralysis of the wrist and fingers can be distinguished clinically and electrically. Stimulation of the radial nerve above the elbow should yield extension of the wrist, fingers, and thumb. Furthermore, with stabilization of the metacarpophalangeal joints in extension, the proximal and distal interphalangeal joints should be actively and easily extended in a posterior interosseous nerve paralysis. Lack of extension of these two terminal digital joints would suggest a hysterical or volitional condition. These two terminal joints are extended by the median and ulnar nerves innervating the intrinsic muscles when the metacarpophalangeal joints are stabilized in extension.[36, 49]

RETURN OF FUNCTION.   The following case gives some insight into the upper limit to which one may expect return of function of this purely motor posterior interosseous nerve. A 6-year-old boy developed a typical spontaneous paralysis of the posterior interosseous nerve which lasted for 1 year. He was unable to extend the fingers or thumb of his left hand (Fig. 34*A* and *B*). His wrist dorsiflexed in a radial direction, and he had normal sensation throughout his hand. There was no history of trauma or injury or evidence of a space-occupying lesion about the elbow, nor was there any systemic cause for the localized paralysis. Surgical exploration of the radial

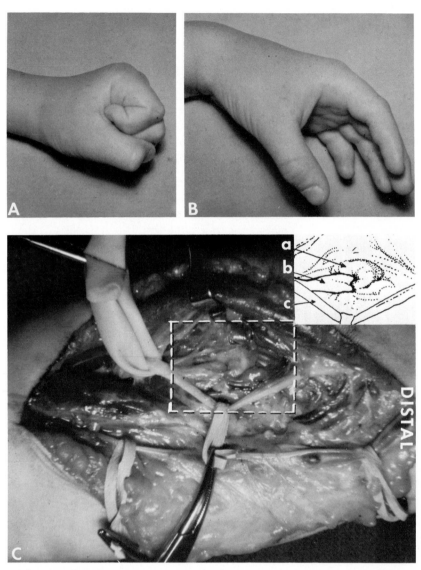

Figure 34.   *A* and *B*, Spontaneous posterior interosseous nerve paralysis of one-year's duration with inability to extend the fingers and thumb of the left hand. *C*, The posterior interosseous nerve is edematous just proximal to where it enters the arcade of Frohse. This arch is thickened and snug about the nerve. (Inset key: a, arcade of Frohse; b, posterior interosseous nerve; c, superficial radial nerve.)

Illustration continued on opposite page

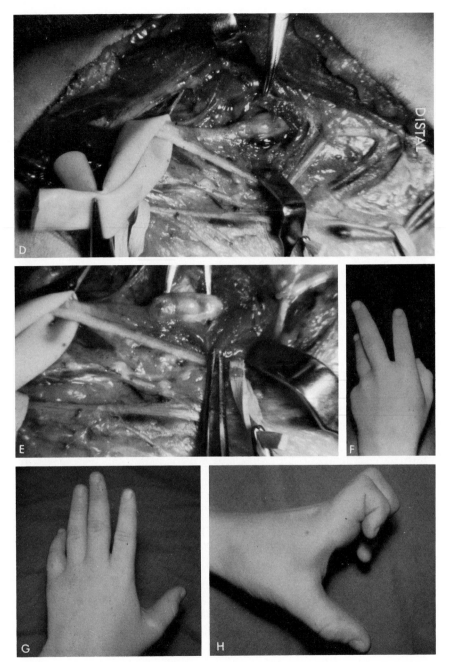

Figure 34 *Continued.* *D* and *E*, Upon decompression of the nerve a pseudoneuroma of the posterior interosseous nerve was found. *F*, *G*, and *H*, Gradual return of extension of the digits at the metacarpophalangeal joint and thumb occurred.

nerve and its major divisions at the elbow revealed that the posterior interosseous nerve was edematous just proximal to where it entered the arcade of Frohse (Fig. 34C). This arch was thickened and snug about the nerve (Fig. 34D). Upon decompression of the nerve a pseudoneuroma lesion was noted (Fig. 34E).

The recovery pattern was of particular interest. As was noted preoperatively, dorsiflexion occurred in a radial direction. After the operation the wrist was first noted to be dorsiflexed in a neutral position, and eventually even in ulnar deviation, indicating reinnervation of the extensor carpi ulnaris. Within 4 months the index and long fingers extended fully at the metacarpophalangeal joints (Fig. 34F–H). At 7 months after neurolysis the thumb, ring finger, and little finger extended fully.

An important feature of this case indicates what can be expected in predicting return of function. Despite 1 year of total paralysis complete return of function ensued, the pseudoneuroma remaining in place. Had the compression continued for a longer period of time, an irreversible fourth degree neural lesion, a neuroma-in-continuity, most likely would have resulted. Mulholland[58] described a lesion so produced as a "fibroma." It appears that following total paralysis of this nature one can expect a motor nerve to regain its function after up to 18 months of nerve compression. The case reported by Goldman et al.[25] supports this opinion.

The time factor is of importance in helping the clinician to decide if primary tendon transfer would be the procedure of choice over exploration of the nerve. In dealing with total paralysis of the nerve, 18 months appears to be the maximal length of time in which return of function can be expected with release of the nerve. Beyond that time, release of the nerve will not restore function of the paralyzed extensors.

This case also provides important insight into electromyographic information, which should be helpful in the management of similar problems. Surgical exploration had not been carried out for 12 months because the posterior interosseous nerve still conducted impulses and had a normal conduction time across the elbow, even though total clinical paralysis was present. An expert electromyographer had concluded that these findings indicated that reinnervation was going to occur. However, after a year there was no clinical improvement in spite of repeated electrical studies, which revealed normal latency of the posterior interosseous nerve across the elbow. Re-evaluation of the conduction curve revealed the probable cause for the misinterpretation to be the presence of a few functioning neural fibers, which resulted in normal conduction time values. A plateau-type curve was the unusual feature suggesting that progressive distal summation of electrical excitation of the muscle had spread through the muscle fibers rather than down the main nerve trunk (Fig. 35). I believe that if clinical or electrical

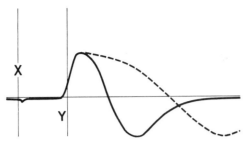

Figure 35.   The nerve conduction studies revealed a plateau-type prolonged evoked response (the dotted line curve). However, there is a normal latency measurement across
the elbow because the XY time (in msec) was not affected. This electrical finding when
present should help confirm the pathology present.

function of the nerve has not returned within an 8- to 12-week period,
exploration of the nerve is indicated.

     This opinion is confirmed by a recent unusual case of posterior
interosseous nerve paralysis which developed in a lymphedematous arm
of a 70-year-old white female. She had had a mastectomy, including an
axillary dissection, for breast carcinoma some 9 years earlier. The paralysis
was present for 2 months. Six months prior she had fallen, sustaining a soft
tissue injury of the forearm with ecchymosis and additional swelling which
required hospitalization. She informed me that she had not had any
fractures, and roentgenograms of the limb did not reveal any new or old
osseous abnormality. There was no evidence of recurrent or metastatic
disease. The hand presented a typical posterior interosseous nerve paralysis with wrist dorsiflexion in a radial deviation and with a lack of extrinsic
extensor function in all the digits (Fig. 36A and B). Sensation was intact.
Exploration of the nerve revealed a constriction of the posterior interosseous nerve at the level of the proximal edge of the tendinous portion of
the supinator (Fig. 36C). No pseudoneuroma or "fibroma" of the nerve
was found. Three months later return of function of the nerve was
noted.

     This case suggests that pathological pressure on the nerve precedes
any fibrosis of the nerve seen in long-standing cases. It appears that
the time lag produces the varying pathology, from constriction of the
nerve to pseudoneuroma and subsequent localized "fibroma." This is a
neuroma-in-continuity, a fourth degree nerve lesion. Beyond 18 months
of total paralysis neurological surgical procedures are disappointing.

     Spontaneous partial posterior interosseous nerve paralysis has a
better prognosis for recovery following prolonged compression. As long
as functioning axons are demonstrated clinically, surgical intervention
consisting of external and internal neurolysis can restore function even
beyond 18 months of paresis of the nerve. This is documented by the case

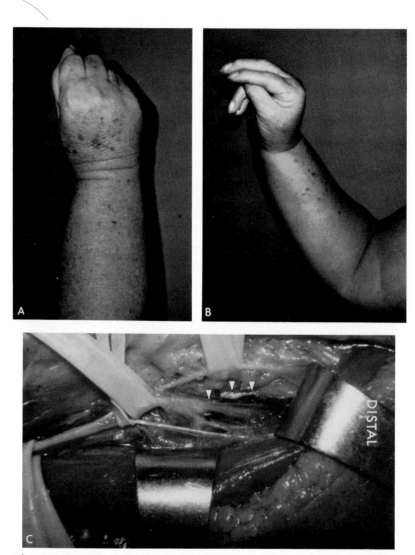

Figure 36. *A* and *B*, The wrist dorsiflexion is in radial deviation. All the digits lack the function of the extrinsic extensors innervated by the posterior interosseous nerve. *C*, The posterior interosseous nerve was constricted (single arrow) at the proximal edge of the tendinous portion of the supinator (double arrow).

of a 48-year-old physician who had a 3 year history of pain in the proximal forearm and progressive inability to extend the thumb or the long, index, and ring fingers. When I first examined him he could extend the little finger only slightly and had a weak extensor carpi ulnaris (Fig. 37A and B). At surgery, the posterior interosseous nerve was identified proximal to the supinator. A dorsoradial proximal forearm surgical approach was used to develop the interval between the extensor digitorum communis and the extensor carpi radialis brevis. The plane was defined to the lateral epicondyle. The elbow was flexed, and the posterior interosseous nerve identified and found not to be compressed at this level. The arcade of Frohse was not thickened. The nerve was traced distally. The superficial head of the supinator was split. At its distal end a 1.5 cm. fibrous band crossed and compressed the nerve (Fig. 37C and D). An external and internal neurolysis was performed, utilizing the operating room microscope, and multiple funiculi with small pseudoneuromata were found (Fig. 37E). The medial funiculi were less involved in the compression. This correlated with the basic internal funicular pattern and the clinical findings. The extensor carpi ulnaris and the extensor digiti quinti funiculi are located medially in the posterior interosseous nerve. With recovery there was progressive improvement, beginning in the tenth postoperative week. By the end of 1 year there was recovery of complete extension of the digits and thumb and neutral dorsiflexion of the wrist (Fig. 37F).

This demonstrates that partial compression lesions of the posterior interosseous nerve can recover motor function well beyond the time limits observed with complete lesions — well beyond 18 months. Here, the partial paralysis had existed for 3 years.

Not all cases of posterior interosseous nerve paralysis require surgical exploration to recover function[38] as exemplified by the following case. A 55-year-old waiter who suffered a spontaneous, painless onset of paralysis of the posterior interosseous nerve involving the extensor of the thumb and fingers (Fig. 30) improved completely after his arm was immobilized in a sling for 4 weeks. When he was last seen 7 years after recovery, there was no recurrence nor development of any systemic disease affecting peripheral nerves. His case may have been an example of nerve compression related to the arcade of Frohse.

During excision of the radial head the nerve is particularly vulnerable to injury.[81] I have seen a 20-year-old girl with a complete posterior interosseous nerve paralysis 4 weeks after radial head excision (Fig. 38A and B). The proper surgical plane between the anconeus and the extensor carpi ulnaris was utilized. The joint was opened and the soft tissues were said to have been "widely" retracted. Postoperatively the patient was found to have developed a complete paralysis. There was no evidence of electroneuromyographic recovery 5 weeks postoperatively. However, on clinical examination, there was increased muscle tenderness on direct com-

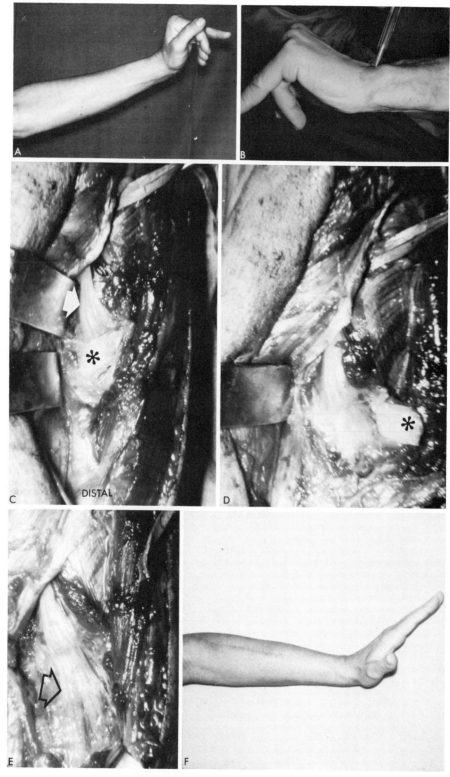

Figure 37.   *See legend on opposite page.*

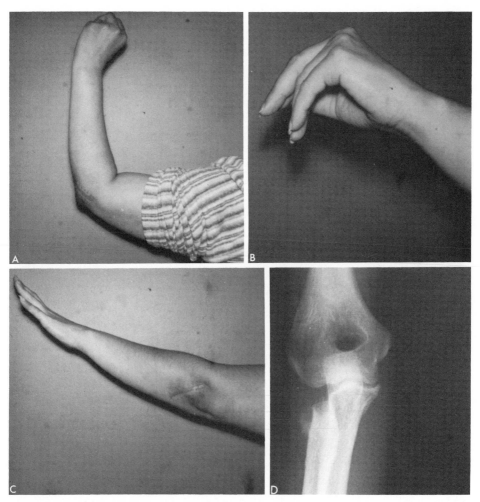

Figure 38.   *A* and *B*, A 20-year-old girl 4 weeks after removal of a comminuted radial head fracture with a complete posterior interosseous nerve paralysis. The fingers and thumb cannot extend at the metacarpophalangeal joints and the wrist extends in a marked radial direction. *C*, At twelve weeks following surgery, spontaneous complete recovery of function of the muscles innervated by the posterior interosseous nerve has occurred. *D*, Roentgenogram 12 weeks after surgery reveals the radial head removed. In addition, there is abundant periostitis of the neck of the radius.

Figure 37.   *A*, A 48-year-old physician with a 3 year history of incomplete ability to extend the fingers and thumb of his left hand. *B*, He can extend only the little finger partially. The extensor carpi ulnaris (at end of pen) functioned but was paretic. *C*, The posterior interosseous nerve (arrow) had initially been identified proximal to its entrance between the two heads of the supinator (at the level of the rubber band). It was traced through this muscle. At the distal end of the supinator a 1.5 cm. fibrous band (asterisk) crossed and compressed the nerve. *D*, The fibrous band (asterisk) was released from its lateral aspect and was flapped medially. *E*, An external and internal neurolysis was performed. Small pseudoneuromas were noted. *F*, There was progressive return of function one year after operation.

pression of the extensor muscles, greater in the involved forearm than in the other. This finding persisted until reinnervation of the muscles at 10 weeks. By 12 weeks there was full recovery (Fig. 38C). Roentgenograms reveal absence of the radial head with excessive periosteal calcification of the neck of the radius (Fig. 38D).

This case indicates that not all posterior interosseous nerve paralyses following radial head excision require surgical exploration. Pain on direct compression of the recovering paralyzed muscles is a helpful prognostic sign, a positive muscle Tinel sign. Nevertheless, even with this sign, if there had not been clinical or electrical recovery by 12 weeks surgical exploration would have been necessary.

Compression of the posterior interosseous nerve becomes a distinct possibility when a fibrous arch of Frohse is present, especially if it is thick and the space for the nerve is narrow. Edema of the adjacent structures, neoplasm, or inflammatory swelling may compress the nerve against the hard unyielding edge of the arch. A ganglion,[7] bursa,[1, 59] lipoma,[11, 55, 63, 67, 90, 95] radial head fracture,[5, 81] aneurysm,[19] Monteggia fracture-dislocation,[44, 56, 77, 79] and dislocation of the elbow have been reported to be responsible for just such a compression.

Paralysis of the posterior interosseous nerve has also been reported in association with rheumatoid disease of the elbow.[48, 51, 54, 56] It is usually secondary to the rheumatoid synovitis that encroaches upon the nerve at the level of the arcade of Frohse. Inability to extend the fingers as a result of nerve paralysis must be distinguished from rupture of the extensor tendons at the wrist level resulting from rheumatoid granulation tissue invading the tendons and rubbing of the tendons against bony prominences. The pathological process can be identified by electromyographic evaluation, by direct muscle stimulation, and by the clinical tenodesing test. If the tendons are ruptured the digits will not extend dynamically when the wrist is flexed. In posterior interosseous nerve paralysis the digits will extend on wrist flexion because the tendons are in continuity. The paralysis can be partial, and the examiner must have a high degree of suspicion and an awareness of the need for differential diagnosis.[54] On occasion, the posterior interosseous nerve paralysis associated with rheumatoid arthritis of the elbow will subside with intra-articular steroid therapy, only to recur after the passage of a considerable period of time (2 years).[51] Permanent recovery followed combined neurolysis, synovectomy and excision of the radial head.

The age of the patient does not affect the prognosis regarding return of function of the posterior interosseous nerve.[42] If neurolysis is done within the 18 month lag period, return of function can be expected even in the elderly. The following example illustrates this. A 68-year-old woman was seen 7 weeks after a comminuted displaced fracture of the radial head with paralysis of the posterior interosseous nerve. There was no clinical or electrical sign of recovery. Exploration of the posterior interosseous nerve was undertaken through an anterior approach. A fibrous band corresponding to the arcade of Frohse was found. At the time of release, the underlying compressed posterior interosseous nerve was found to be pale and flattened, with adhesions to the adjacent soft tissues (Fig. 39). The branches of the recurrent radial vessels in the area were found to be thrombosed. Six weeks later, a return of function of the muscles innervated by the posterior interosseous nerve was evident. Three months after surgery, return of strength to all the muscles innervated by this nerve was noted.

Another patient, 65 years of age, was seen 8 weeks after a markedly comminuted radial head fracture associated with a posterior interosseous nerve paralysis. There was no clinical or electrical return of nerve function. About 12 weeks following neurolysis of the posterior interosseous nerve through an anterior approach, and removal of fragments of the comminuted radial head, function of the nerve was restored.

EARLY CLINICAL SIGNS OF RECOVERY FROM COMPLETE POSTERIOR INTEROSSEOUS NERVE PARALYSIS.   The patient is asked to abduct the thumb of the involved hand while the examiner palpates just distal to the ulnar styloid on the dorsoulnar aspect of the wrist for contraction of the extensor carpi ulnaris. When this muscle is re-innervated, its tendon becomes taut under the examiner's fingers.

Furthermore, with recovery of the extensor carpi ulnaris, the wrist, which ordinarily dorsiflexes in a radial direction when there is complete posterior interosseous nerve paralysis, now dorsiflexes in a less radial direction.

Two basic facts, one anatomical and the other physiological, explain these signs. The motor end plates of the extensor carpi ulnaris are closest to the nerve trunk of all the muscles innervated by the posterior interosseous nerve. Wallerian degeneration and subsequent regeneration of axons to this muscle usually take the shortest time. Kinesiologically, there is synergistic activity between antipulsion of the thumb and contraction of the extensor carpi ulnaris (Fig. 40). This relationship between the two was described by Duchenne.[20] It is an interesting observation because abduction of the thumb is basically a median nerve–innervated function, whereas the extensor carpi ulnaris is supplied by the posterior interosseous nerve, which is a major branch of the radial nerve.

LACERATION INJURIES.   The posterior interosseous nerve can be injured anywhere from its origin at the main radial nerve trunk at the level of the radiocapitellar joint down to its motor end plates.[52, 57] Most frequently, it is injured in the proximal third of the forearm. This nerve can be repaired successfully even at its point of division at the lower border of the supinator muscle.

A typical case is one in which a 12-year-old boy on July 4th, 1965, sustained a laceration at the junction of the proximal and middle third of the right forearm (Fig. 41A). It was caused by an empty can which was

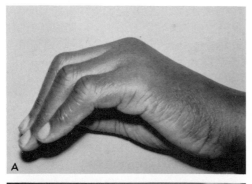

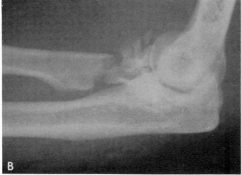

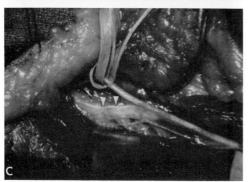

Figure 39. *A* and *B*, A 68-year-old black woman had sustained a comminuted fracture of the radial head 7 weeks earlier. She had a posterior interosseous nerve paralysis. *C*, The compressed posterior interosseous nerve (arrows) was found to be pale and flattened with adhesions to the adjacent soft tissues.

Figure 40. Antipulsion of the thumb is synergistic with contraction of the extensor carpi ulnaris.

hurled by a firecracker explosion. He was unable to extend the metacar-pophalangeal joints of the fingers because of paralysis of the extensor digitorum communis, extensor proprius and extensor digiti quinti mus-cles (Fig. 41B). When the carpometacarpal and metacarpophalangeal joints of the thumb were stabilized in extension, the patient was unable to extend the distal joint of the thumb due to paralysis of the extensor pollicis longus (Fig. 41B). Immediate exploration of the wound revealed a complete laceration of the extensor digitorum communis muscle, but what was even more important, all five terminal branches of the posterior interosseous nerve were found to be severed. Each of the branches was repaired (Fig. 41D and E). Full return of finger extension occurred within 4 months after nerve repair. The thumb had normal extension at all joints (Fig. 41F and G).

It is important to note that the recurring branch to the common extensor muscles (as previously described), which innervates the proximal 40 per cent of the muscle, should be repaired. Otherwise, there will be weakness in extension of the middle two digits. The index and fifth fingers, which have double musculotendinous units, will have full exten-sion but the middle two digits will display a weakness, especially when the wrist is fully dorsiflexed. This was noted in another patient who had a similar injury. In this case the weakness of extension of the two middle digits was disturbing enough to the patient to warrant tendon transfer to the extensor digitorum communis to improve the dexterity of the fingers.

It should be noted that the motor nerve branch to the extensor carpi radialis brevis descends a short distance within the radial nerve adjacent to the superficial radial nerve. It has a long extraneural course along the medial border of its muscle before its entry. Therefore, if it is lacerated it can be repaired in acute injuries. Stookey (1922)[80] had noted this. The extensor carpi radialis brevis is the chief neutral strong dorsiflexor of the wrist. Its functional recovery contributes to normal wrist stability in the long axis of the forearm. It should be emphasized that a closed injury with paralysis of the posterior interosseous nerve should be treated conserva-tively during the initial 8 to 12 weeks because in the majority of cases spontaneous return of function occurs. However, a laceration of the posterior aspect of the forearm not associated with a fracture in which a posterior interosseous nerve paralysis is present should be explored immediately after the injury. Primary neurorrhaphy will most likely be necessary. A compound fracture of the proximal radius with a posterior interosseous nerve paralysis would best be explored and debrided with care and the status of the nerve evaluated. Most of the time, the nerve is just contused; however, if the nerve has been severed, it can be repaired after reduction and fixation of the fracture of the radius, if the wound, time lapse, and skin coverage permit. Otherwise, the nerve should be

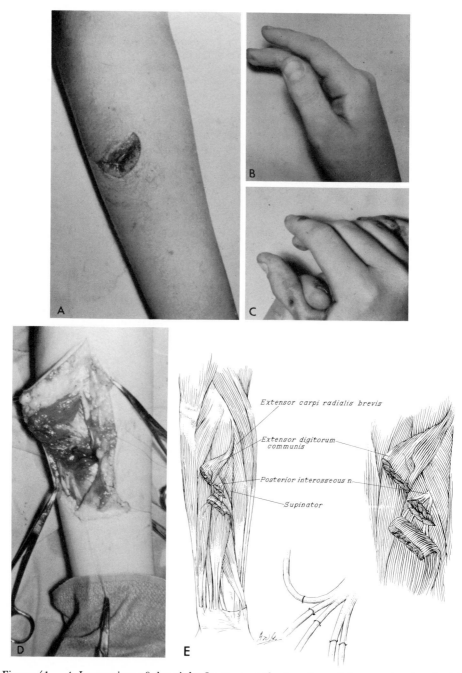

Figure 41.   *A*, Laceration of the right forearm at the junction of the proximal and middle third portions caused by explosion of a firecracker under an empty can. *B*, The fingers cannot extend fully at the metacarpophalangeal joints. *C*, The terminal phalanx of the thumb cannot extend when its metacarpophalangeal joint is in extension. *D* and *E*, The five terminal branches of the posterior interosseous nerve were found to be severed. They were repaired with fine sutures and a funicular type reapproximation.

Illustration continued on opposite page

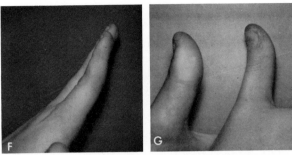

Figure 41   *Continued.*   F and G, Four months after the funicular repair the thumb could extend fully at all its joints and the digits extended completely at the metacarpophalangeal joints.

repaired secondarily. Thus, the status of the nerve will be known and procrastination can be avoided.

FRACTURE AND DISLOCATION INJURIES.   The posterior interosseous nerve can be involved in fractures of the shaft of the radius at the junction of the proximal and middle third portions. The following case is of a 12-year-old girl who sustained multiple fractures of the right upper extremity, segmental fractures of both bones of the forearm (Fig. 42A), and a fracture of the surgical neck of the humerus and clavicle. There were abrasions of the dorsum of the right forearm. All the fractures were closed. This was accompanied by a typical paralysis of the posterior interosseous nerve (Fig. 42C). An attempt to treat the patient by closed reduction was unsuccessful. To avoid a cross-union, an intramedullary Steinmann pin was introduced into the ulna for stabilization. The nerve was not explored. Six weeks after the operation the paralysis cleared, as noted by return of full finger and thumb extension (Fig. 42D). No cross-union developed, and the segmental fracture of the radius healed satisfactorily (Fig. 42B). The greatest part of the rotation of the forearm (70 per cent) was preserved.

In another case, a posterior dislocation of the elbow without a radial fracture with a posterior interosseous nerve paralysis did not show improvement within 12 weeks following reduction. Exploration of the nerve was necessary. Thrombosed vessels were found crossing and constricting the nerve, which explained the persistent dysfunction. Six weeks after the neurolysis a partial return of function was noted, and full recovery occurred 3 months later.

In another group of fracture-dislocations of the elbow (the Monteggia lesion), four cases of posterior interosseous nerve paralysis were seen in children (Fig. 43A–D). All were reduced by closed methods immediately after injury. The nerve recovery occurred either within 3 days or by 8 weeks after injury.[77]

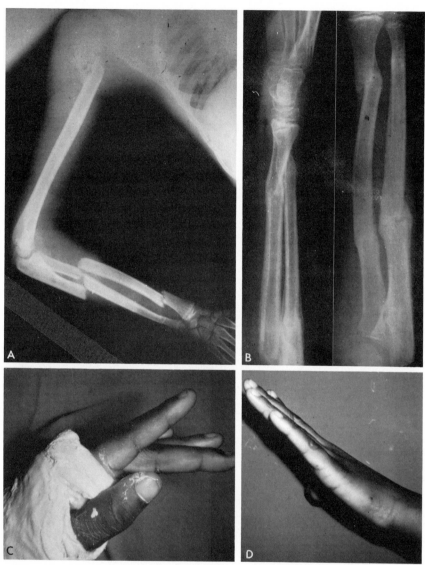

Figure 42. *A*, A 12-year-old black girl sustained segmental fractures of both bones of the forearm, of the surgical neck of the humerus, and of the clavicle. *C*, She had a typical posterior interosseous nerve paralysis. *B*, The segmental fractures of the forearm healed satisfactorily after open reduction of the ulna. *D*, Six weeks after the operative procedure the paralysis cleared spontaneously, as noted by return of full finger and thumb extension.

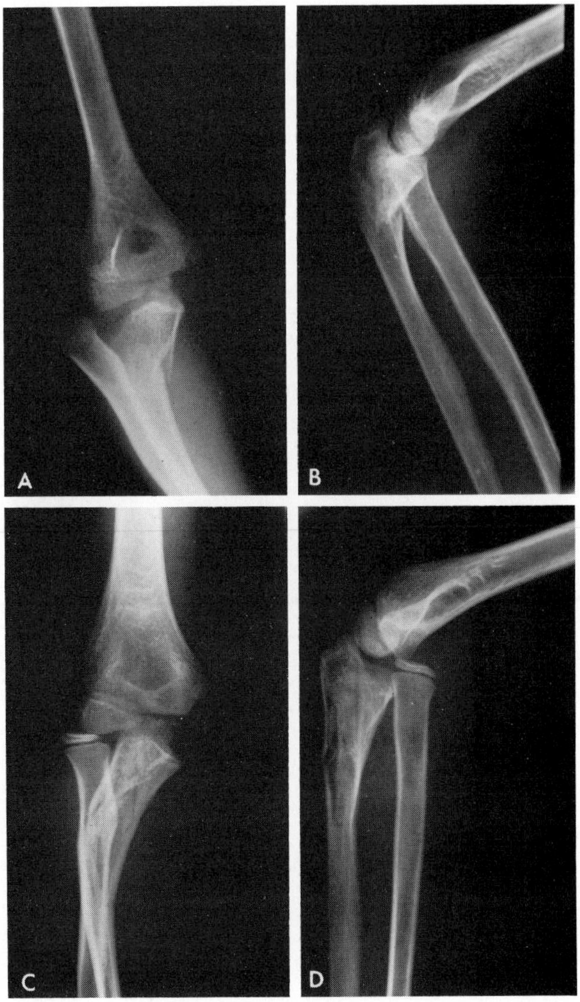

Figure 43.   *A* and *B*, Anteroposterior and lateral roentgenograms of a flexion type Monteggia lesion. The fracture-dislocation was posterolateral. *C* and *D*, Anteroposterior and lateral roentgenograms of an extension-type Monteggia fracture-dislocation of the elbow. The radial head is dislocated anterolaterally. All the posterior interosseous nerve paralyses associated with the Monteggia lesion encountered in children were associated with lateral displacement of the radial head.

In adults, most closed Monteggia fracture-dislocations associated with posterior interosseous nerve paralysis respond to conservative measures within a few weeks after the ulna is reduced (usually with internal fixation), with the radial head reduced by supinating the forearm. However, if function of the posterior interosseous nerve does not return within 8 weeks, exploration of the nerve is necessary.

The nerve can be injured with other nerves of the forearm — none is exempt. Posterior interosseous nerve paralysis can occur simultaneously with anterior interosseous nerve paralysis. I have seen a cardiologist who had this combined neural lesion following fracture of the midshaft of the radius and subsequent plating fixation. He had the classic posterior interosseous nerve motor extensor loss of the digits and thumb, and was unable to flex the terminal phalanx of the thumb. Sensation was intact throughout the hand. It was not clear when the combined paralysis developed. He was said to have had an inordinate amount of preoperative pain. One month after surgery, when I first examined the patient, there was early clinical evidence of recovery of extension. Gradually the medial digits extended at the metacarpophalangeal joints. It took 4 months for recovery of the extrinsic long flexors and extensors of the thumb and index fingers to occur (Fig. 44A–D).

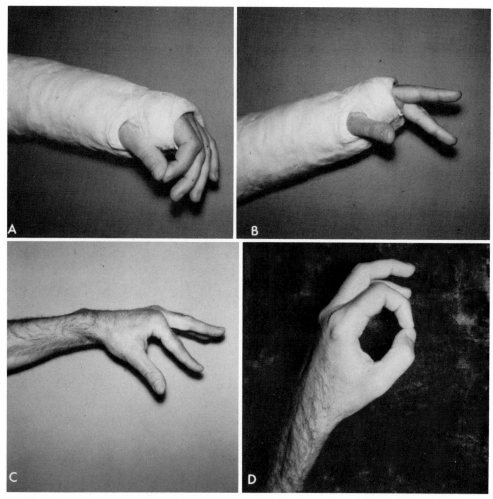

Figure 44.   *A*, One month after plating in fracture of the shaft of the left radius the terminal phalanx of the thumb does not flex. The terminal phalanx of the index finger can flex. The patient has a partial anterior interosseous nerve paralysis. *B*, He cannot extend the thumb and digits at the metacarpophalangeal level. The partial extension of the index finger is produced by the plaster, which is partially supporting this joint. He has a complete posterior interosseous nerve paralysis as well as a partial anterior interosseous nerve paralysis. *C*, A month later there has been partial recovery of the posterior interosseous nerve, as noted by return of extension of the long, ring, and little fingers at the metacarpophalangeal joint. The index finger and thumb recovered extension power one month later. *D*, Four months after injury the patient could flex the terminal phalanx of his thumb normally.

The incomplete nature of the anterior interosseous nerve paralysis was a good prognostic sign. Especially when there was associated early progressive recovery of posterior interosseous nerve function. The neural lesions were probably a mechanical traction-compression injury of both the anterior and posterior interosseous nerves. Prognosis for recovery of the injury to the anterior interosseous branch of the median nerve also was good. The lesion was partial—only the flexor pollicis longus was paralyzed, while the flexor profundus muscles of the index finger and long fingers functioned, permitting flexion of the terminal phalanges of these digits. Inability to flex or extend the terminal phalanx of the thumb should immediately suggest to the examiner that more than one nerve or major nerve branch is affected.

BULLET WOUNDS.   Bullets of low or high velocity produce different effects in passing through the extensor region of the forearm. In civilian life the low velocity bullet injury produces a transient paralysis which usually responds without extensive debridement. In contrast, in military injuries sustained in combat in which there is excessive destruction to the adjacent muscular tissue and long segments of the nerve, reconstruction by tendon transfers after the wound is healed is more appropriate.[2, 52] There is similar extensive muscle and nerve damage as a result of civilian shotgun injuries of the extensor surface of the proximal forearm. Here, too, tendon transfers are indicated frequently.

COMPRESSION LESIONS.   Volkmann's ischemic process of the forearm, which most frequently causes entrapment of the median and ulnar nerves, can, in addition, cause compression of the posterior interosseous nerve. One such case required prompt release of all three nerves. The posterior interosseous nerve entrapment was at the arcade of Frohse (Fig. 45A and B). The patient responded well to release of all three nerves (Fig. 17).

A bursa arising from the bicipital region has been described as being large enough to cause combined lesions of the posterior interosseous nerve and the median nerve. In 1863, Dr. D. H. Agnew,[1] in an article, "Bursal Tumour Producing Loss of Power of Forearm," which appeared in the American Journal of Medical Sciences, presented the specimen and made the following remarks:

> The tumour was about the size of a hickory nut, and was situated at the bend of the left arm, on the inner side of the tendon of the biceps muscle. Patient a female. It had been growing slowly for two years, was elastic to the feel, and exquisitely sensitive. The power of the flexor muscles of the fingers and thumb, and the extensors of the forearm generally, was so much diminished as to render the limb comparatively useless. The tumour made but little show externally, being bound down by the deep fascia of the arm, and in flexion and extension of the arm appeared to follow the movements of the tendon of the biceps muscle. I regarded it as of bursal origin, and accounted for the muscular phenomena from other contiguity or attachment to the nerves inclosing the muscles involved.
>
> In its removal an incision was made through the skin directly over the growth, the

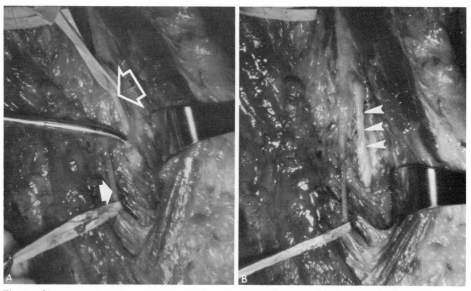

Figure 45. *A*, Left forearm in 19-year-old boy with Volkmann's ischemic contracture of 3 weeks' duration. The posterior interosseous branch of the radial nerve (open arrow) is traced to thickened arcade of Frohse (under hemostat). The superficial radial nerve (solid arrow) is also identified. *B*, After release of the arcade of Frohse, the posterior interosseous nerve is noted to be narrowed in the region (arrows).

median basilic vein pushed aside, the laminae of cellular tissue divided on a director, and the bicipital aponeurosis opened, when the tumour came into view, when, on a careful inspection, it was found to have the median nerve investing its anterior surface spread over it in a membranous form, and likewise adherent. This was carefully dissected away, and, on turning out its deep surface, a similar, though not so extensive, connection was found to exist with the posterior interosseous nerve. A single narrow prolongation alone retained the growth, which descended beneath the tendon of the biceps muscle to the bursa situated between it and the tubercle of the radius.

The history of its formation might doubtless be stated as follows: A few fibres supporting the bicipital bursal membrane had yielded under some strain, allowing the latter to bulge through, and to increase gradually in size by the accumulation of fluid. Subsequently, the tumor became solidified by inflammatory products becoming organized.

The tumour contained no fluid contents, but consisted of formation of fibrous or connective tissue in various stages of development. The recovery was most satisfactory, the lady having very soon regained the use of all the muscles implicated.

Various types of soft tissue tumors that can produce compressive lesions of the posterior interosseous nerve have been seen; I have treated several cases. In one a bicipital bursa was the cause of a posterior interosseous nerve paralysis (Fig. 46). In another case, a lipoma was the causative tumor (Fig. 47). In a third case a large fibroma was found to arise from the soft tissues adjacent to the arcade of Frohse (Fig. 48). The vital structures in this area must be identified prior to excising a lesion here. In a fourth case a hemangioma arising from the recurrent radial vessels (Fig.

Text continued on page 127

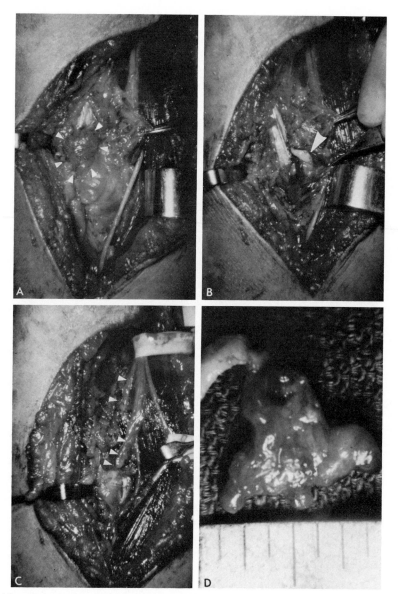

Figure 46. *A*, An enlarged bicipital bursa of the right forearm is noted. *B*, The arrow indicates a large rice body in the bursa. The biceps tendon is seen proximal to and extending into the region of the bursa. *C*, The bursa has been excised, and the posterior interosseous nerve is visualized (three small white arrows). The superficial radial nerve is in the rubber band to the right. The terminal portion of the main radial nerve trunk is in the Penrose proximally. The nerve to the extensor carpi radialis brevis is indicated by the two small white arrows. *D*, The bursa with its rice body is 2.5 cm. in width.

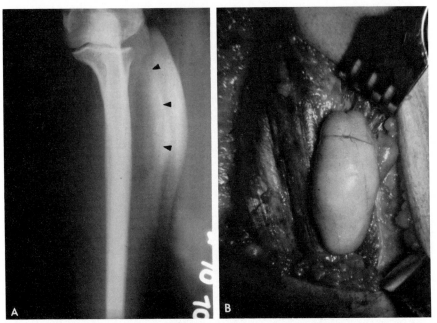

Figure 47.   A lipoma adjacent to the neck of the radial head casts a radiolucent shadow (*A*). It can produce a posterior interosseous nerve paralysis in this location. *B*, The appearance of the lipoma at the time of its removal.

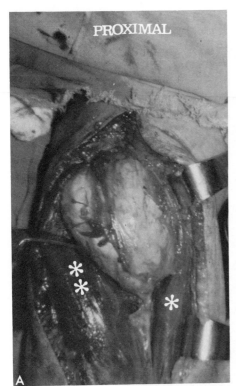

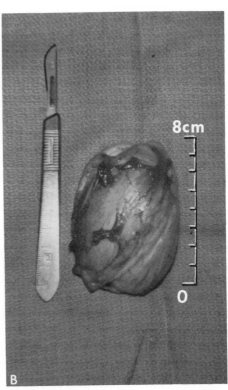

Figure 48.   A, A large benign soft tissue tumor in a right elbow arose from the fibrous soft tissue in the region of the arcade of Frohse. The internervous plane between the brachioradialis (**) and the pronator teres (*) has been developed. B, An 8 cm. fibroma was removed.

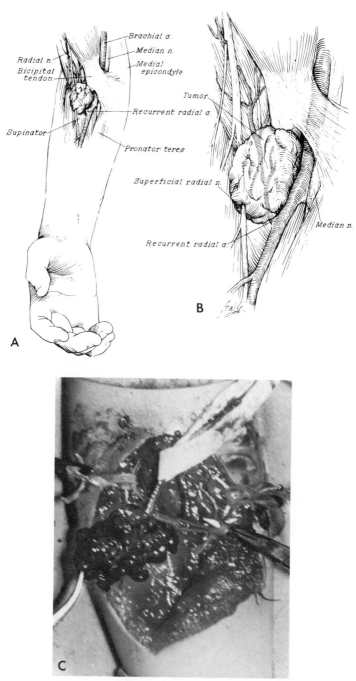

Figure 49.   A hemangioma arising from the recurrent radial vessels presented clinically with hypesthesia of the dorsal and volar aspects of the thumb due to the combined compression of the superficial radial nerve and the median nerve.

49) presented with unusual findings. A palpable mass was noted on the radial side of the antecubital fossa. There was hypesthesia of the dorsum of the thumb as well as the palmar aspect due to combined superficial radial nerve compression and partial median nerve compression. In this instance, following removal of the tumor, sensation returned in 3 weeks. The rapid return of sensory function indicates that the neural injury was a neurapractic lesion.

Finally, three cases of posterior interosseous nerve palsy have been reported as a manifestation of isolated paralysis in the newborn.[17] The condition has been ascribed to abnormal positioning *in utero*. The infants were immobilized in padded plaster splints with the wrist and fingers in extension. All had full return of function by the seventh week of life. This condition must be differentiated from congenital absence of the extensor muscles of the forearm.

Tardy Posterior Interosseous Nerve Palsy

Tardy posterior interosseous nerve paralysis can occur but with much less frequency than is observed with the ulnar nerve at the elbow. I have observed this lesion, which presented initially as a partial paralysis, in a 28-year-old female who was able to extend her little finger at the metacarpophalangeal joint only. Gradually, over a 2 year period, she became unable to extend her thumb, index, long and ring fingers (Fig. 50). The remainder of her hand had normal function, and her wrist extended satisfactorily. There was a scar on the dorsum of her proximal forearm: as a child she had had osteomyelitis of the radius which had required

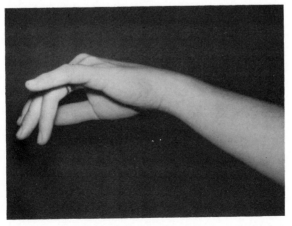

Figure 50.   Tardy partial posterior interosseous nerve paralysis due to an old osteomyelitis of the proximal radius which occurred 20 years before. Only the little finger can extend at the metacarpophalangeal joint.

saucerization. As has been demonstrated by Strachan and Ellis,[81] in the proximal 4 cm. of the forearm, the posterior interosseous nerve moves 1 cm. or more medially relative to the radius on pronation. Surgical neurolysis of the posterior interosseous nerve was performed, and the nerve was found to be fixed to the periosteum of the radius from the level of the neck through the upper third. Over a period of 20 years several factors had developed which probably produced the palsy: there was fixation of the nerve to the radius; the radius had grown throughout childhood and adolescence; and, with repeated pronation of the forearm, traction injury to the posterior interosseous nerve probably occurred. There was, in addition, some compression factor in the pathogenesis of this lesion because the arcade of Frohse was noted to be thickened. For recovery of this type of neural lesion, which is secondarily due to osteomyelitis, release of the arcade of Frohse alone at the proximal end of the supinator is insufficient. Neurolysis of the posterior interosseous nerve throughout its full course in the proximal forearm is necessary. The nerve should be traced through the entire supinator.

Tardy palsy of this nerve has also been reported in a patient with a long-standing (38 years) Monteggia fracture-dislocation.[44] The deformed radial head was dislocated in a dorsoradial direction. Similar prolonged subtle mechanical injury to the nerve as well as aging probably caused the paralysis. Following neurolysis of the posterior interosseous nerve, and excision of the radial head, there was significant neural recovery.

TENDON TRANSFER FOR NONFUNCTIONING OR IRREPARABLE POSTERIOR INTEROSSEOUS NERVE PARALYSIS.   In irreparable complete paralysis of the posterior interosseous nerve, several solutions may be considered. The transfer described by Riordan[68] has become my favorite and has produced excellent end results in managing this problem. The flexor carpi ulnaris is transferred around the ulnar border of the forearm and inserted into the extensor digitorum communis tendons just proximal to the extensor retinaculum. For the thumb, the extensor pollicis tendon is first detached from its muscle and withdrawn from its tunnel adjacent to Lister's tubercle. It is then transferred in a straight line, following the direction of the abductor pollicis brevis and extensor pollicis brevis. The palmaris longus tendon is the usual new motor source. Its tendon is detached distally, transferred around the radial border of the forearm, and sutured to the rerouted proximal end of the extensor pollicis longus tendon at the proper tension. This latter transfer produces combined extension of the distal and proximal phalanges of the thumb and abduction of the first metacarpal. When the palmaris longus is absent, the extensor carpi radiális longus is an alternate motor. In this instance, the flexor carpi radialis must be maintained to flex and stabilize the wrist.

For a different management, the flexor carpi ulnaris can be transferred to the finger extensors and long thumb extensor, and the palmaris longus to the abductor pollicis longus and extensor pollicis brevis. Again the flexor carpi radialis is left for flexion of the wrist.

Boyes[8] described a procedure in which the flexor superficialis muscles of the long and ring fingers are passed through the interosseous membrane for extension of the fingers and thumb, and the flexor carpi radialis is transferred to the abductor pollicis longus and extensor pollicis brevis. This has the advantage of leaving the flexor carpi ulnaris functioning. The normal wrist axis of function (dorsoradial to volar ulnar) would be maintained.

At times after a posterior interosseous nerve repair, only partial recovery may be obtained. In addition, late untreated cases present a loss of function of some of the muscles innervated by the posterior interosseous nerve. In this instance it is a matter of determining which digit or digits lack metacarpophalangeal joint extension. If the functional loss warrants reconstruction, any one of several motors is available for transfer, such as the flexor carpi ulnaris, a flexor superficialis, a radial wrist extensor, the flexor carpi radialis, and even the brachioradialis. The choice of tendon transfer is influenced by what has to be restored, the presence of function of the extensor carpi ulnaris, and the strength of the proposed active motor, as well as other factors, such as the condition of the tissue bed in line with the course of the transplanted tendons, skin coverage, mobility of the joints, and cooperativeness of the patient.

The Radial Tunnel Syndr

Resistant Tennis Elbow Due to Posterior Interosseous Nerve Compression

Entrapment of the posterior interosseous nerve as a cause of tennis elbow has been suggested for almost two decades. Capener,[12, 13] Somerville,[76] and recently Roles and Maudsley[69] have proposed the association. Three sites of compression in the radial tunnel have been noted. The tendinous origin of the extensor carpi radialis brevis and the arcade of Frohse were the most frequent sites. The other site was at the level of the radial head, where adhesions have been observed.[69] In one case, I have seen a radiohumeral bursa anterior to the radial head in juxtaposition to the posterior interosseous nerve (Fig. 51). It is indeed conceivable that the adhesions observed on occasion with resistant tennis elbow due to posterior interosseous nerve compression are the result of radiohumeral bursitis. The pathology is usually related to the extensor carpi radialis brevis tendinous origin or the proximal thickened edge of the superficial head of the supinator.

The pain usually occurs anteriorly over the head of the radius in the course of the nerve and its branches, and can be clinically reproduced in three ways:

(The Hand: diagnosis & indications: churchill - Livingstone)

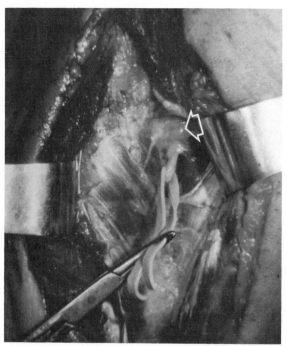

Figure 51.   The posterior interosseous nerve with a small bursa (arrow) adjacent to it is visualized in a right elbow. There had been an additional larger radiohumeral bursa which had ruptured in the course of the dissection. This collapsed bursa is seen just distal to the intact bursa overlying the nerve. Surgery had been performed for resistant tennis elbow. The patient has been asymptomatic following the neurolysis and removal of the bursae.

1. By direct pressure along the nerve anterior to the radial head.

2. By resisting extension of the long finger, especially with the elbow in extension.

3. By inflating a tourniquet below systolic pressure on the arm, producing venous congestion.

The associated signs that are observed include weakness of grip of the hand, paresthesia in the skin of the dorsum of the thumb, pain on resistance to supination of the forearm, pain on passive stretch of the extensor muscles, and restriction of the last few degrees of extension of the elbow.

Electroneuromyographic studies can help to confirm the neural compression etiology of the resistant tennis elbow. Fibrillations in the muscles innervated by the posterior interosseous nerve, or conduction delay across the elbow along this nerve, will corroborate the diagnosis. Unfortunately, the correlation is not always present. Thus, it requires good insight and clinical acumen to make the diagnosis of entrapment of the posterior

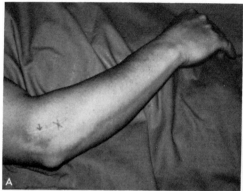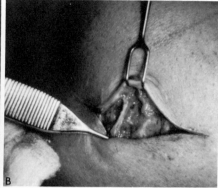

Figure 52.   *A*, Patient had had prior surgery for right lateral epicondylitis but he had post-operative pain which was of neuromatous quality. He had a positive Tinel sign (at X). *B*, Neuroma of the posterior cutaneous nerve of the forearm is seen at end of the forceps. The patient's pain was relieved following removal of the neuroma and allowing the proximal end of the nerve to retract into a fatty bed after it was tied with a fine nylon suture.

interosseous nerve as a cause of tennis elbow. Furthermore, lateral epicondylitis due to tendinous pathology adjacent to the epicondyle and entrapment of the posterior interosseous nerve can co-exist. Management of both causes for the patient's complaint are necessary before the symptoms are relieved.

Persistent pain about the lateral aspect of the elbow following soft tissue surgery for lateral epicondylitis need not be related to compression of the posterior interosseous nerve, for the pain can be the result of a postoperative neuroma of the posterior cutaneous nerve of the forearm (Fig. 52*A* and *B*). This sensory nerve passes close to the lateral epicondyle and is vulnerable to damage when surgery is performed in this region. The nerve arises from the radial nerve at the proximal portion of the spiral groove of the humerus and traverses the lateral aspect of the arm to supply the posterior region of the forearm.

One must suspect that this neuroma is present when the type of postoperative pain has changed in quality and characteristics to that of a neuroma. A positive Tinel sign is present in or just proximal to the scar. In addition, there is an area of anesthesia or hypesthesia of the skin of the dorsoradial aspect of the forearm distal to the scar. This strip of skin suffering sensory disturbance is anatomically smaller than expected because of overlap from nerves of adjacent intact forearm skin, from the posterior division of the musculocutaneous nerve, and from the medial cutaneous nerve of the forearm. The posterior cutaneous nerve of the forearm can be preserved during extensive soft tissue surgery on the dorsoradial aspect of the forearm (Fig. 53*A*–*C*).

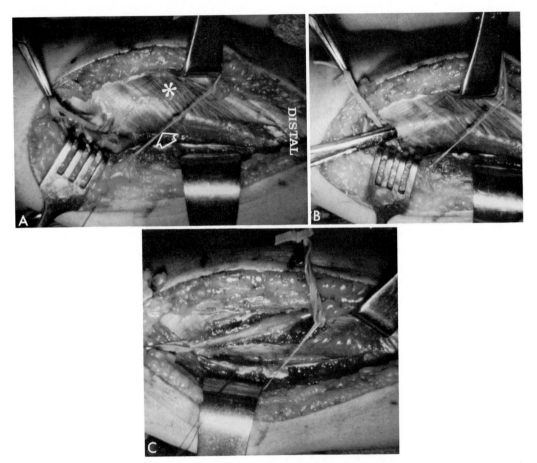

Figure 53. *A*, In a left forearm the interval between the extensor digitorum communis and the extensor carpi radialis brevis has been developed. The posterior interosseous nerve (rubber band) is seen under the proximal edge of the superficial head of the supinator (asterisk). The posterior cutaneous nerve of the forearm has been preserved (arrow). *B*, The hemostat is passed under the superficial head of the supinator in the course of the posterior interosseous nerve. *C*, Note that the posterior interosseous nerve has been exposed throughout its course through the supinator.

Variations of the Posterior Interosseous Nerve and the Superficial Radial Nerve

POSTERIOR INTEROSSEOUS NERVE.   Several variations of the posterior interosseous nerve have been delineated. Harburger[30] described the nerve supply to the abductor pollicis longus and extensor pollicis brevis and a muscle variant with a special supply to the extensor proprius of the middle finger which penetrated the superficial head of the supinator close to its distal end, rather than with the full posterior interosseous nerve from under the cover of the superficial head. Krause[37] and von Luschka[47] described the motor branch to the abductor pollicis longus and extensor pollicis brevis, extensor pollicis longus, and extensor indicis proprius passing superficial to the superficial head of the supinator, while the remaining major portion of the posterior interosseous nerve, supplying the extensor digitorum communis, extensor digiti quinti proprius, and extensor carpi ulnaris, follows its usual course.

Dr. Kaplan and I performed a dissection on a specimen with an anomalous muscle, the extensor brevis manus indicis, an accessory extensor indicis, which arose from the dorsum of the distal radius and the lunate and inserted into the extensor hood mechanism of the index finger. Its nerve supply was found to be a continuation of the branch of the posterior interosseous nerve which innervated the extensor pollicis longus (Fig. 54B). Interestingly enough, we have seen a physician who had a lump on the dorsum of the hand in the identical location of the accessory muscle (Fig. 54A). When this swelling was stimulated electrically there was noted prompt extension of the index finger. In the past, swellings of this type have been confused with a ganglion of the dorsum of the hand.

Typically, in adults the supinator is 5 cm. broad, and the distance from the point of division of the nerve at the distal end of the supinator to the point of penetration of the corresponding muscle is as follows:

Extensor carpi ulnaris — 1.25 cm.
Extensor digitorum communis — 1.25–1.8 cm.
Extensor digiti quinti — 1.8 cm.
Abductor pollicis longus — 5.6 cm.
Extensor pollicis brevis — 6.5 cm.
Extensor indicis proprius — 6.8 cm.
Extensor pollicis longus — 7.5 cm.

Variations in these distances are to be expected and are noted by Sunderland.[83] However, the basic pattern of innervation of the extensor carpi ulnaris and extensor digitorum communis muscles before the outcropping muscles is relatively constant.

These measurements have clinical significance. A hand afflicted with a posterior interosseous nerve paralysis usually dorsiflexes in a radial direction. On occasion, the wrist can dorsiflex more neutrally. If a varia-

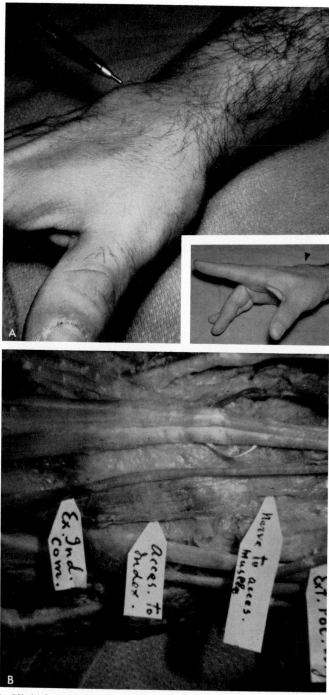

Figure 54. *A*, Clinical appearance of the accessory extensor indicis, the extensor brevis manus indicis muscle. It presents a diagnostic problem with the much more frequent dorsoradial ganglion. *B*, Right anatomical dissection specimen of the dorsum of the distal forearm and hand. Note that the nerve to the accessory extensor is one of the terminal branches of the posterior interosseous nerve.

tion of the insertion of the radial extensors of the wrist exists, the hand can dorsiflex without radial deviation in complete posterior interosseous nerve paralysis. The extensor carpi radialis longus can have a tendinous attachment to the brevis tendon, or there can be an insertion of the longus, not only to the base of the second metacarpal but also to the third, which produces this functional variation with this neural lesion.

After a successful neurorrhaphy or neurolysis of this nerve the earliest clinical sign of impending recovery is the ability of the wrist to dorsiflex in a neutral, or even ulnar, direction. This indicates returning function to the extensor carpi ulnaris and to some extent to the extensor digitorum communis. The synergism between antipulsion of the thumb and contraction of the extensor carpi ulnaris as an early test of posterior interosseous nerve recovery has been noted (Fig. 40). The fingers and thumb usually regain extensor power a few months later.

On extremely rare occasion, as noted by Linell,[45] the motor branch to the extensor carpi radialis longus may arise from the posterior interosseous nerve and penetrate the supinator muscle to reach its destination. In this instance a lesion or compression of the posterior interosseous nerve may present with not only dropped fingers but also a dropped wrist. The hand would have no sensory abnormalities nor would there be a paralysis of the brachioradialis muscle. The latter observation localizes the lesion to the elbow region rather than the arm.

According to Rauber (1868) the anterior interosseous nerve is divided into three long branches. The main branch supplies the flexor pollicis longus, the flexor profundus muscles to the index and long fingers, and the pronator quadratus. The other two branches pass adjacent to the interosseous membrane where they innervate this membrane and the periosteum of the radius and ulna. Some of these branches penetrate the interosseous membrane to communicate with terminal branches of the posterior interosseous nerve (#17 in Fig. 55). In the distal forearm a terminal branch of the main anterior interosseous nerve branch posterior to the pronator quadratus can pass through a foramen in the interosseous membrane to anastomose with branches of the posterior interosseous nerve (#28 in Fig. 55). This latter communication can occur at the distal border of the interosseous membrane. This is a potential pathway for median nerve to radial nerve interchange of neural fibers. Furthermore, the median nerve, at times, can have funiculi destined to innervate intrinsic muscles of the hand. These fibers usually pass through the Martin-Gruber communication from the median nerve to the ulnar nerve, but some of them may reach the intrinsic muscles via the posterior interosseous nerve. This is probably another example of neural plexification that occurs throughout the entire peripheral nervous system.

This variant nerve pathway may have clinical significance. When present it helps explain function of the intrinsic muscles in a hand when

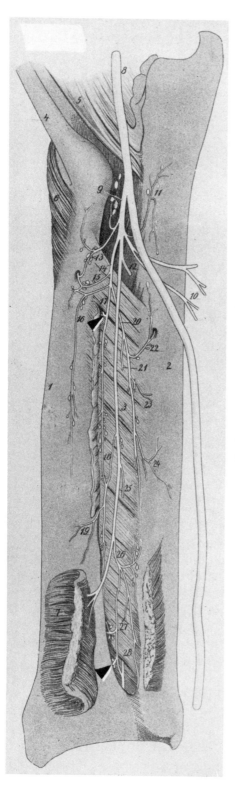

Figure 55. A potential communicating pathway, between the median and radial nerves (black arrows) through the interosseous membrane (17) and near its distal end (28), is illustrated in Rauber's detailed description of the anterior interosseous nerve. (From Augustus Rauber: Ueber die Nerven der Knochenhaut, und Knochen des Vorderarmes und Unterschenkels. Munich, C. Fritsch, 1868.)

the ulnar nerve has been completely severed. Further clinical study is necessary to clarify this possible pathway—median nerve to posterior interosseous nerve through the interosseous membrane.

SUPERFICIAL RADIAL NERVE. Variations of the superficial radial nerve have been described. At times the entire superficial radial nerve may be absent. Appleton[3] described one such case in which the musculocutaneous nerve was found to supply the autonomous zone of the thumb. In several specimens and clinical cases, we have seen the musculocutaneous

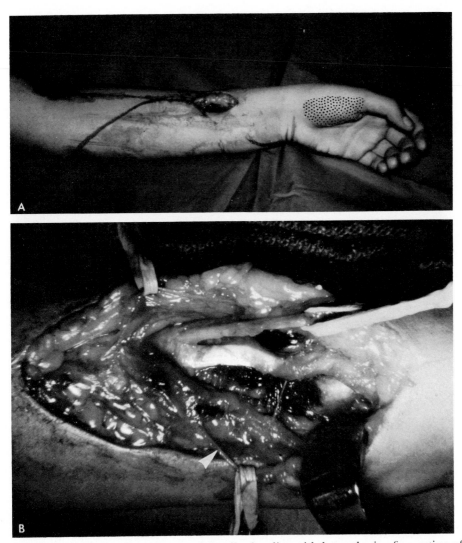

Figure 56. *A*, Compound fracture of the distal radius with hypesthesia of a portion of the thenar eminence (dotted area). *B*, Enlarged view of the wound reveals that the traumatized nerve was the terminal branch of the musculocutaneous nerve (arrow). The undamaged superficial radial nerve is in the rubber band.

nerve coming far down into the hand to supply the anterior volar aspect of the thumb in the region of the first metacarpal between the sensory region of the median palmar cutaneous nerve area and the more dorsal superficial radial autonomous zone (Fig. 56). The superficial radial nerve can supply the thenar eminence, which is usually innervated by the palmar cutaneous branch of the median nerve, and the volar aspect of the thumb. Thus, it is possible for an injury to the superficial radial nerve to produce numbness or anesthesia of both the dorsal and volar aspects of the thumb. In Appleton's specimen the radial nerve continued on as the posterior interosseous nerve. The superficial radial nerve was absent; the dorsum of the thumb was supplied by the enlarged ulnar dorsal cutaneous nerve. The musculocutaneous nerve has been found to supply this same dorsal region of the thumb, that is, the "autonomous" radial sensory zone.

Knowledge of this variation can be clinically significant. I have treated a patient who had a prior open reduction of a fracture of the lower third of the radius. He had severe pain in the surgical scar and numbness of the dorsum of the thumb. It was suspected that a superficial radial neuroma was present. At surgery, several neuromata of the anterior division of the musculocutaneous nerve were found. Search for the superficial radial nerve adjacent to the radial artery deep to the brachioradialis failed to reveal this nerve (Fig. 57).

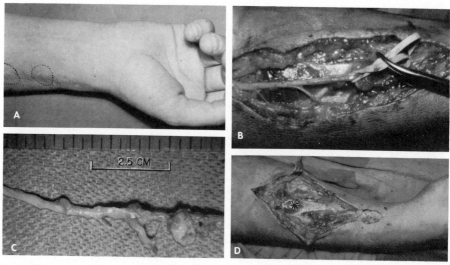

Figure 57. *A,* The two dotted areas center on the region of the positive Tinel sign in the scar. *B,* In the rubber band is the anterior division of the musculocutaneous nerve in the distal forearm in situ. *C,* Two neuromata are seen in the pathological specimen. *D,* No superficial radial nerve was found deep to the brachioradialis (asterisk) or in the soft tissues at the musculotendinous junction of this muscle. The musculocutaneous nerve supplied the area of the thumb said to be "autonomous" for the superficial radial nerve.

On rare occasion, the superficial radial nerve can supply the entire dorsum of the hand. Learmonth[43] reported an anatomical specimen in which the entire dorsal cutaneous branch of the ulnar nerve was absent. The region usually innervated by the ulnar nerve was supplied by an enlarged superficial radial nerve, which had additional branches. This variation is of clinical significance in evaluating the level of the ulnar nerve lesion. High ulnar nerve lesions ordinarily present with sensory loss of the dorsoulnar aspect of the hand in addition to the usual ulnar sensory loss in the fifth digit and half of the fourth digit, along with intrinsic muscle paralysis. Low ulnar lesions have normal sensation in the region of hand innervated by the ulnar dorsal cutaneous nerve in the presence or absence of this anatomical variation. The localization of the ulnar nerve lesion by clinical sensory findings alone would not be accurate in the presence of this variation. Electromyographic conduction studies will help localize the lesion. The presence of this variation in a high ulnar nerve lesion with normal sensation on the dorsoulnar aspect of the hand can then be confirmed by a local anesthetic block of the superficial radial nerve. I have observed this diagnostic problem on two occasions.

The superficial radial nerve may follow an aberrant course. On rare occasions the superficial radial nerve can wind around the brachioradialis muscle at the elbow, passing down the forearm superficial to, rather than deep to, this muscle. Furthermore, when there is a complete fusion of the brachioradialis and extensor carpi radialis longus muscles, then it is possible, as has been reported, that the superficial radial nerve may perforate the fused conjoint tendon in the lower forearm. The superficial radial nerve, then, is a key to the posterior interosseous nerve. The superficial radial nerve can be traced proximally to the radial nerve trunk through the area of partial or complete fusion of the brachioradialis and brachialis muscles. The other two branches are then dissected distally, the posterior interosseous nerve and the motor branch to the extensor carpi radialis brevis thus can be identified easily and safely.

Superficial radial nerve dysfunction by itself has been noted and recorded by Wartenberg.[88] I have seen one boy who had hypesthesia on the dorsum of the right thumb without any history of laceration but with pain in the elbow. There was no paralysis of the posterior interosseous nerve. He responded well to immobilization in a cast, which put the elbow at rest, and he has had no recurrence of the difficulty. The etiology and pathology in this case are not clear.

A hemorrhage in the proximal forearm on the radial aspect can result in a superficial radial neuritis. Fibrosis about this nerve caused by the organized hematoma can be augmented by thrombosis of branches of the anterior and posterior recurrent radial vessels. Persistent pain in the proximal forearm that is associated with localized reproduction of the complaint with percussion along the course of this nerve is diagnostic of

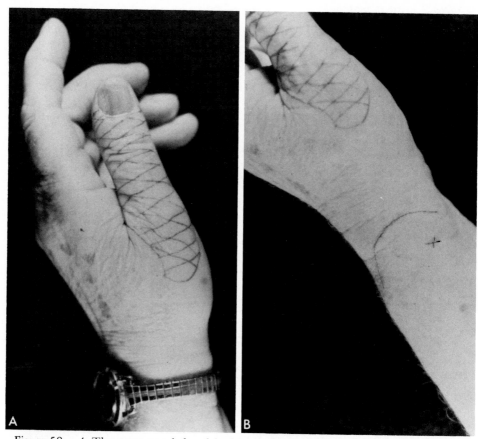

Figure 58.   *A*, The same watch band had been worn continuously for 20 years on the left wrist. In recent months numbness of the dorsum of the thumb (hatched area) developed, as did pain in the wrist. *B*, There was a positive Tinel sign (X) located 1 cm. proximal to the distal end of the radius.

the condition when numbness of the dorsum of the thumb is also present. Neurolysis of the superficial radial nerve may be necessary when conservative measures fail.

Severe spontaneous pain can develop insidiously in the distal forearm. It can be caused primarily by an external compression mechanism involving the superficial radial nerve. It should be suspected when there is a positive Tinel sign adjacent to the radial styloid and there is numbness of the skin of the dorsum of the thumb. In one case, a patient developed these symptoms when she wore the same watch band for 20 years. She had gained weight and had salt and water retention. The tight band caused direct compression of the superficial radial nerve against the unyielding underlying radius (Fig. 58).

The chief of neurosurgery at my community hospital developed identical annoying, and at times distressing, symptoms. He wore the same size operating gloves for 15 years. He too had water retention. The thick, rolled ends of the gloves caused the compression.

In both instances, removal of the offending external circular band relieved the symptoms; however, it took 3 to 4 months for symptoms to subside completely.

The superficial radial nerve can be injured when a cutdown of a vein in the lower forearm is performed. The nerve passes dorsally from under the brachioradialis and becomes subcutaneous about 10 cm. above the radial styloid. Thus, it is particularly vulnerable in this region. In addition, when the extensor carpi radialis brevis tendon is lengthened for a tennis elbow in the Garden procedure, care must be taken not to injure this sensory nerve because the procedure performed is precisely at the level where the superficial radial nerve emerges dorsally from under the cover of the brachioradialis.

Causalgias of the superficial radial nerve have presented problems to many physicians.[46] I have seen patients who have required a cervical sympathectomy because of the sympathetic overflow secondary to a neuroma of this nerve. Sometimes nerve repair can be done successfully. At other times symptoms can be relieved by excising the neuroma and resecting the nerve into a new soft tissue bed. Silastic caps for the end of the severed nerve have been recommended by Frackelton et al.[21] All of these measures have their appropriate indications in the proper cases. For example, if the patient has a large sympathetic overflow or discharge with stiffening of the hand secondary to the superficial radial nerve injury, he may not respond to conservative measures and may require operative sympathectomy, while other patients may do well with excision of the neuroma. In others, removal of the suture and neurolysis where the nerve has been caught in a ligature of a cutdown procedure may solve the problem.

The two major branches of the superficial radial nerve are vulnerable to injury during the operative procedure for deQuervain's disease. The branches are located close to the first extensor compartment. They must be identified and preserved. Furthermore, they should be retracted with care before releasing the abductor pollicis longus and extensor pollicis brevis tendons.

A snug, minimally padded plaster cast which is utilized to maintain a Colles fracture reduced in ulnar deviation can compress a superficial radial nerve branch at the first metacarpal level, especially if there is undue pressure at the distal end of the cast. Permanent numbness on the dorsum of the thumb distal to the compression can result if there is scarring of the skin overlying the superficial radial nerve branches.

Linell[45] has noted that because of the communication between the anterior division of the musculocutaneous nerve and the superficial radial nerve in the lower third of the forearm, lacerations of the superficial nerve in the proximal forearm may not present clinically with sensory manifestations in the hand. The five isolated lacerations of the superficial radial nerve I have seen have presented with anesthesia or hypesthesia of the dorsum of the base of the thumb. Two had considerable pain which required surgical measures.

Interestingly, a young nurse presented initially with symptoms and findings suggested of a recurrent deQuervain's disease of the wrist following successful surgery 3 years earlier. She stated that she had noted residual hypesthesia of the dorsum of the thumb which gave her no difficulty following the initial surgery. Wrist and thumb complaints recurred after a minor injury. After unsuccessful conservative management, surgery revealed a neuroma of one of the branches of the superficial radial which was bound into the residual scar from the previous surgery. A resection of the neuroma with crush and fine tie of the cut nerve branch, bringing the nerve end into normal tissue bed, relieved her "recurrent" deQuervain's disease.

It is of particular interest that a schwannoma of this nerve does not produce pain or sensory disturbance. Frequently, this nerve tumor presents clinically as a painless mass. When it is removed carefully by shelling it out, preserving the splayed axons over the mass, the patient can remain symptom-free postoperatively.

Finally, the superficial radial nerve can be entrapped when this nerve perforates a common brachioradialis and extensor carpi radialis brevis tendon at the junction of the middle and distal thirds of the forearm.[32] Localized neuritic symptoms may develop at the site of this failure of muscle–tendon segmentation.

Variations of the Muscles of the Radial Aspect of the Elbow

SOLITARY HEAD OF THE SUPINATOR.   Quain[72] and Testut[85] do not mention a solitary head as a variation of the supinator muscle. Otenasek[61] reported a solitary head of the supinator, and in his text LeDouble[40] has noted that on occasion "the supinator was reduced to an aponeurotic layer intermixed with a few very pale muscular fibers." He was not aware of it being absent except in association with congenital absence of the radius. Straus[82] believes the supinator to be a distal migration of a more proximal muscle. He suggests that the supinator of mammals is derived from the deeper fibers of the primitive humeroradial extensor that arose from the distal humerus and inserted on the radius.

There have been isolated reports of absence of the superficial head of the supinator muscle. In such instances the posterior interosseous nerve would lie directly on the supinator, not pass through it.

FUSION OF THE BRACHIORADIALIS AND BRACHIALIS MUSCLES.   On occasion there may be a fusion or perhaps a lack of segmentation of the

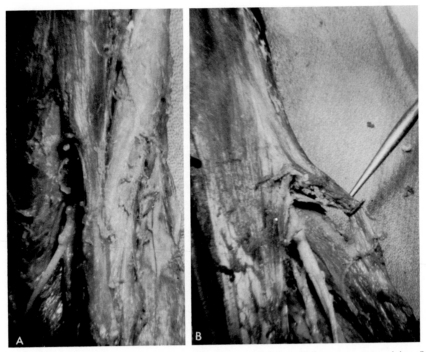

Figure 59.   *A*, A dissected right limb with the superficial radial nerve seen arising from the radial nerve. The plane between the brachioradialis and brachialis is clear. *B*, In this left arm specimen there is partial fusion between the brachialis and brachioradialis muscles (in the hook). The radial nerve with its superficial and posterior interosseous nerve division is noted deep to the partial fusion of the brachioradialis and brachialis.

brachioradialis and brachialis. This may be complete or incomplete. The incomplete fusion is more common than the complete (Fig. 59*A* and *B*).

There are variations of the deep muscles of the extensor group which consist of duplication or accessory muscles or absent muscles.[29]

The extensor brevis manus, an accessory short extensor to the fingers, occurs quite frequently. Sometimes, it is an accessory to the index finger only. It arises from the carpus, and is usually innervated by a terminal branch of the posterior interosseous nerve.

ACCESSORY MUSCLES OF THE ANTEROLATERAL ASPECT OF THE ELBOW. The accessory brachialis (also noted as the brachialis minor), because of its insertion at times into the fascia of the forearm (the lacertus fibrosus), may be troublesome if the surgeon is unaware of its possible occurrence.

The accessory brachioradialis[40] (also known as an intermediary supinator[14] or a reduplicated brachioradialis) is of significance in presenting as an additional structure arising from the lateral condylar ridge of the humerus and inserting on the radius at varying levels from the bicipital

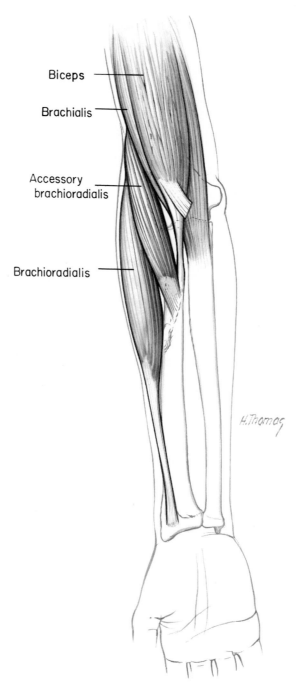

Biceps

Brachialis

Accessory
brachioradialis

Brachioradialis

H. Thomas

Figure 60.   The accessory brachioradialis arises from the distal humerus and inserts into the proximal radius adjacent to the bicipital tuberosity. This variant muscle can originate as far proximally as the deltoid tuberosity of the humerus. It can insert as far distally in the forearm as the lower third of the radius. (Adapted from Wood, J: Proc. Roy. Soc. Lond. *16*:496, 1868.)

tuberosity (Fig. 60), proximally to the radial styloid distally. Its origin can extend proximally on the lateral aspect of the humerus and lateral intermuscular septum to the deltoid tuberosity.[94]

Froment-Rauber Nerve

Innervation of the first dorsal interosseous muscle and the adjacent second and third dorsal muscles may, on occasion, occur from a terminal branch of the posterior interosseous nerve. This was first described by Froment[23] in 1846, and further noted by Rauber[65] in 1865 (Fig. 61). It was mentioned by Shevkunenko (1949),[74] who made similar anatomical findings (Fig. 62).

Bichat,[6] as early as 1802, noted this anastomosis between the terminal branches of the posterior interosseous nerve and the deep branch of the ulnar nerve in the dorsal interosseous muscles of the hand. Hovelaque[33] also notes the Froment-Rauber anastomosis.

In view of the earlier description by Bichat of the anastomosis between the posterior interosseous nerve and the deep branch of the ulnar nerve, perhaps it would be more precise to add the name of Bichat to the eponym, Froment-Rauber interneural communication.

Communicating branches between the median and musculocutaneous nerves in the arm and between the median and ulnar nerves in the

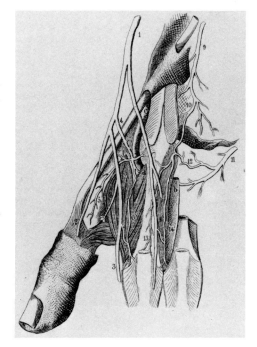

Figure 61. The details of the anastomosis (12) between the terminal branches of the posterior interosseous (9) and the deep branch of the ulnar nerve (11) is seen. There is also a potential anastomosis between the superficial radial nerve (1) and the ulnar nerve (11) in the first and second interosseous muscles. The first dorsal interosseous muscle and adjacent intrinsic muscles can on occasion be innervated by the terminal branches of the radial nerve. (From Augustus Rauber: Vater'sche Korper der Bander und Periostnerven. Inaug. Diss., Munich, 1865.)

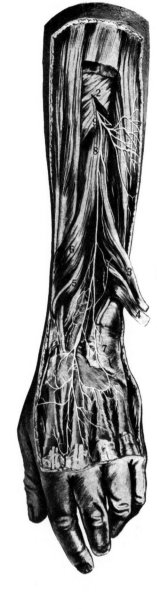

Figure 62. The details of the Froment-Rauber anastomosis are noted over the dorsum of the interosseous muscles. (From V. N. Shevkunenko: Atlas of Peripheral Nervous and Venous Systems. Moscow, Medgiz, 1949.)

forearm have been noted frequently. However, passage of fibers from the ulnar or median nerve through the interosseous membrane has not been reported in man. Straus[82] has noted that in lower reptiles and amphibians such communications through the interosseous membrane are not uncommon. In man, however, it would seem that the most likely proximal course of the Froment-Rauber nerve fiber exchange and crossing path would be at the level of the brachial plexus. Some of the C8–T1 fibers to the intrinsic muscles probably pass distally via the posterior cord to the posterior interosseous nerve rather than through the usual medial cord to the ulnar nerve path. Nevertheless, exchange through the interosseous membrane cannot be entirely ruled out.

OPERATIVE APPROACH TO THE RADIAL NERVE

The radial nerve, and its major branches at the elbow, can be exposed throughout its course in the lower arm and forearm through an incision which begins anteriorly between the brachialis and the brachioradialis in the arm and extends dorsally into the forearm between the extensor carpi radialis brevis and the extensor digitorum communis (Fig. 63). The radial nerve in the lower arm is identified by developing the interval between the

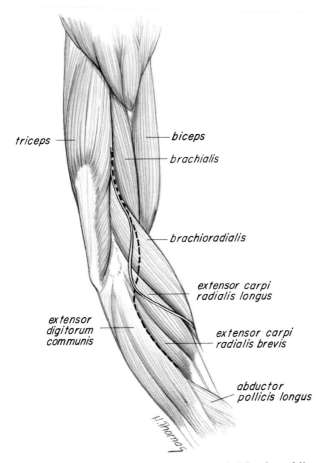

Figure 63.   The muscles of the right forearm are noted. The dotted line represents the incision for complete exploration of the radial nerve and its posterior interosseous branch. The continuous lines outline the incision useful to expose the radial nerve and the proximal half of the posterior interosseous nerve as well as the superficial radial nerve.

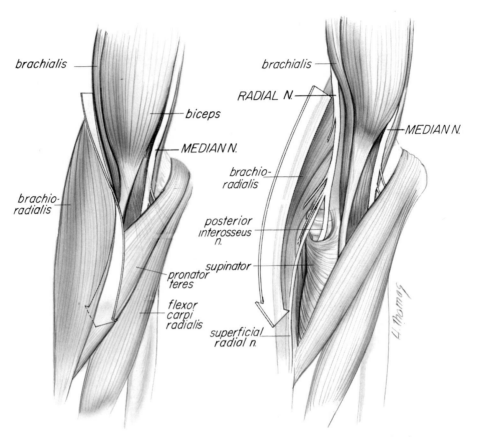

Figure 64.   The radial nerve and its major forearm branches, the posterior interosseous nerve and the superficial radial nerve, are identified by developing anteriorly the interval between the brachioradialis and brachialis in the distal arm. In the proximal forearm the plane continues between the brachioradialis and the pronator teres.

brachioradialis and the brachialis (Fig. 64). On the medial side of the brachioradialis, deep to its fascia, the main trunk of the radial nerve can be identified just proximal to the elbow. It is surrounded by fat and can be traced distally to its bifurcation, the superficial radial nerve and the posterior interosseous nerve in the proximal forearm.

The development of the interval between the extensor carpi radialis brevis and the extensor communis is difficult if one just incises through the aponeurosis near the lateral epicondyle. However, the proper plane can be defined distally and the common longitudinal raphe between these two muscles can be separated by defining the distal interval and dissecting proximally to the lateral epicondyle (Fig. 65). The supinator muscle is then visualized in the depth of the wound.

The muscular fibers of the supinator pass obliquely from its origin at the lateral epicondyle of the humerus and the adjacent ulna to its insertion

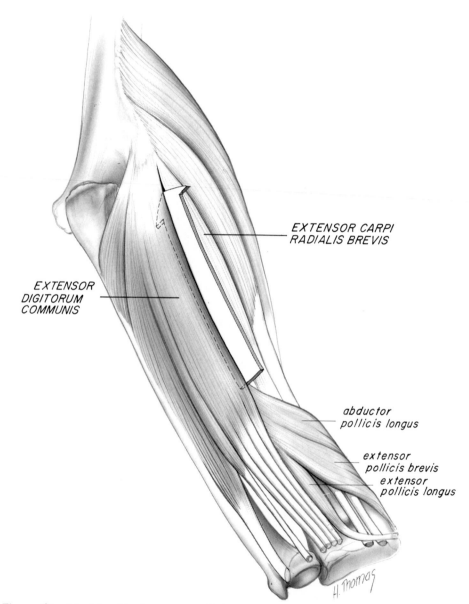

EXTENSOR CARPI
RADIALIS BREVIS

EXTENSOR
DIGITORUM
COMMUNIS

abductor
pollicis longus

extensor
pollicis brevis

extensor
pollicis longus

H. Thomas

Figure 65.   To identify the course of the posterior interosseous nerve through the
supinator it is necessary first to open the plane between the extensor carpi radialis brevis
and the extensor digitorum communis.

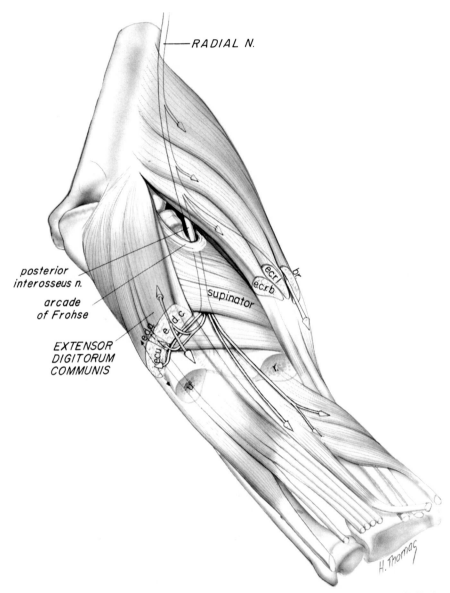

RADIAL N.

posterior
interosseus n.

arcade
of Frohse

EXTENSOR
DIGITORUM
COMMUNIS

supinator

ecrl
ecrb

br

edc

ecu

edq

r

u

H. Thomas

Figure 66. After the internervous plane between the extensor carpi radialis brevis (e.c.r.b.) and the extensor digitorum communis (e.d.c.) is developed the posterior interosseous nerve is identified just proximal to the arcade of Frohse. It can be traced through the supinator, where distally its multiple terminal branches can be visualized (br. = brachioradialis, e.c.r.l. = extensor carpi radialis longus, e.c.u. = extensor carpi ulnaris, r. = radius, u. = ulna).

on the proximal radius. At the lower end of the supinator, the terminal branches of the posterior interosseous nerve are seen. They appear like the branches of the cauda equina dividing in a fanlike fashion (Fig. 66). There is one important anatomical relationship at this point. The proximal 40 per cent of the extensor digitorum communis muscle is innervated by its motor branch from the posterior interosseous nerve, which has a recurrent proximal course. The plane between the supinator and the extensor digitorum communis should not be cleared with blunt force because this would endanger the motor supply to the extensor digitorum communis, extensor digiti quinti and extensor carpi ulnaris. Thus, the more superficial muscles of the extensor group — the extensor digitorum communis, the extensor digiti quinti and the extensor carpi ulnaris — must get their supply from the plane of the deeper located posterior interosseous nerve and should be defined with care, since these motor branches pass between the superficial and the more deeply located extensor muscles. The motor branches of the posterior interosseous nerve which supply the deeply located outcropping muscles (the abductor pollicis longus, the extensor pollicis brevis, the extensor pollicis longus and the extensor indicis proprius) stay on the deep musculoskeletal plane of the forearm.

On the dorsal surface of the proximal forearm, the posterior interosseous can be identified passing deep to the arcade of Frohse. Its course is in a straight line, passing at the neck of the radius, in a dorsoulnar direction deep to the superficial head of the supinator muscle. If the posterior interosseous nerve is identified proximally, its path can be traced distally within the supinator. Thus, any lesion within the region of the supinator can be identified clearly (Fig. 53).

The posterior interosseous artery and vein do not travel with their companion nerve in the proximal third of the forearm (Fig. 19B). These vessels join the nerve at the level of the distal end of the supinator. Since the deep head of the supinator extends more distally than the superficial head, in the region where the posterior interosseous nerve divides, the vessels have not as yet joined the posterior interosseous nerve. The vessels do so at the distal edge of the deep head of the supinator. The brachioradialis and the extensor carpi radialis longus and brevis muscles are left undisturbed in the posterior approach.

For lesions in the region of the arcade of Frohse, only the proximal half of the exposure may be necessary. In such a case, the skin incision is modified so that the interval between the brachioradialis and the brachialis in the lower third of the arm is followed. At the elbow joint the incision is brought radially and is curved so that it avoids crossing the flexion crease of the elbow; it then sweeps down the anterior part of the forearm, paralleling the anterior border of the brachioradialis. The curved portion of the skin incision is dissected down to the level of the deep fascia. The musculocutaneous nerve is identified and preserved.

The skin is elevated, with its underlying fat, at the level of the retaining deep fascia of the forearm. The cephalic vein can be preserved and retracted with a rubber dam; one crossing vein may have to be sacrificed to give complete visualization of the area. The musculocutaneous nerve penetrates the fascia deep to the biceps muscle, 3 to 4 cm. proximal to the elbow joint. The fascia over the medial aspect of the brachioradialis is divided longitudinally. The superficial radial nerve is identified posterior to the brachioradialis muscle and is traced proximally to the radial nerve. It should be noted that the superficial radial nerve runs within the fascial compartment of the brachioradialis. This relationship is important because sometimes the brachioradialis and the brachialis are fused and the proximal interval cannot be identified clearly. In this instance, by tracing the superficial radial nerve proximally to the main radial nerve trunk, the fusion can be separated safely without endangering the vital structures in this region.

After the main radial nerve trunk is identified, the posterior interosseous nerve and a motor branch to the extensor carpi radialis brevis are clearly visualized. From the anterior approach, the posterior interosseous nerve can be traced through the proximal half of the supinator without difficulty. The crossing vessels running at right angles to the superficial radial nerve in the proximal arm must be ligated (Fig. 67). They usually are

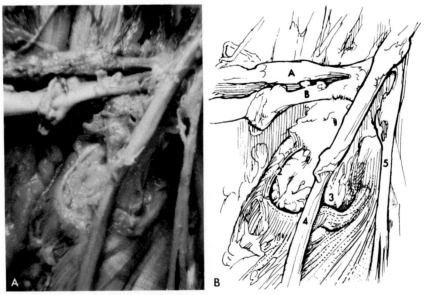

Figure 67.   Dissection specimen, left arm. Note the size of the recurrent vessels (A and B) seen coursing at a right angle to the superficial radial nerve (4). The arcade of Frohse (2) and the posterior interosseous nerve (3) are seen deep to the superficial radial nerve (4) and the nerve to the extensor carpi radialis brevis (5).

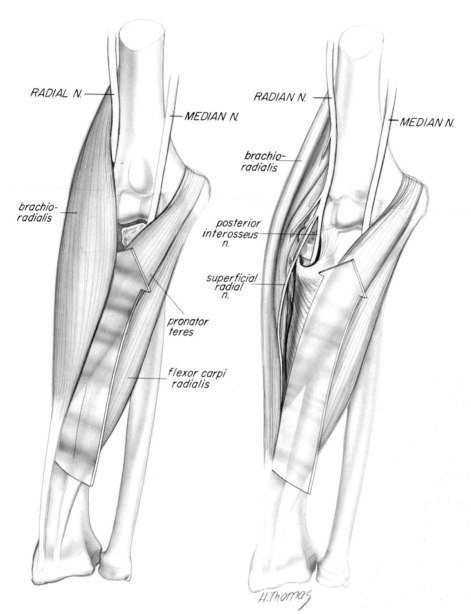

Figure 68.   When anomalies exist on the radial side of the proximal forearm the super-ficial radial nerve is the key to accurate exposure. It is traced proximally to the radial nerve and then distally to its major branches at the elbow level, the posterior interos-seous nerve and the motor branch to the extensor carpi radialis brevis. The interval developed is between the brachioradialis and the pronator teres.

in an anterior and posterior leash. These vessels are a part of the radial recurrent anastomosis.

Where the brachioradialis and brachialis interval cannot be defined clearly the key to safe exposure of this region is the superficial radial nerve (Fig. 68). It can be traced proximally through the region of the muscular fusion or variation. To visualize the posterior interosseous nerve completely requires, in addition, exposure of the distal half of the supinator muscle. To do so, the interval between the extensor carpi radialis brevis and the extensor digitorum communis is developed. The proximal and distal portions of the posterior interosseous nerve are identified, and any lesion between, such as a lipoma, a ganglion or a lacerated nerve in the region of the supinator, can be identified clearly.

BIBLIOGRAPHY

1. Agnew, D. H.: Bursal Tumor Producing Loss of Power of Forearm. Amer. J. Med. Sci., 46:404–405, 1863.
2. Albritten, F., Jr.: The Surgical Repair of the Deep Branch of the Radial Nerve. Surg. Gynecol. Obstet., 82:305–310, 1946.
3. Appleton, A. B.: A Case of Abnormal Distribution of the N. Musculocutaneous, with Complete Absence of the Ramus Cutaneus N. Radialis. J. Anat. Physiol., Third Series, 46:89–94, 1911–1912.
4. Barber, K. W., Jr., Bianco, A. J., Jr., Soule, E. H., and MacCarty, C. S.: Benign Extramural Soft Tissue Tumors of the Extremities Causing Compression of Nerves. J. Bone Joint Surg., 44A:98–104, 1962.
5. Bateman, J. E.: Trauma to Nerves in Limbs. Philadelphia, W. B. Saunders, 1962.
6. Bichat, X.: Traité d'Anatomie Descriptive. Paris, Brosson and Gabon, XI, 1802, p. 270.
7. Bowen, T. L., and Stone, K. H.: Posterior Interosseous Nerve Paralysis Caused by a Ganglion at the Elbow. J. Bone Joint Surg., 48B:774–776, 1966.
8. Boyes, J. H.: Bunnell's Surgery of the Hand. 5th Ed., Philadelphia, Lippincott, 1970, pp. 418–419.
9. Brash, J. C.: Neuro-Vascular Hila of Limb Muscles. Edinburgh and London, E. and S. Livingstone, 1955.
10. Bryan, F. S., Miller, L. S., and Panijaganond, P.: Spontaneous Paralysis of the Posterior Interosseous Nerve: A Case Report and Review of the Literature. Clin. Orthop., 80:9–12, 1971.
11. Campbell, C. S., and Wulf, R. F.: Lipoma Producing a Lesion of the Deep Branch of the Radial Nerve. J. Neurosurg., 11:310–311, 1954.
12. Capener, N.: Posterior Interosseous Nerve Lesions. Proceedings of the Second Hand Club. J. Bone Joint Surg., 46B:361, 1964.
13. Capener, N.: The Vulnerability of the Posterior Interosseous Nerve of the Forearm. J. Bone Joint Surg., 48B:770–773, 1966.
14. Cirio, J. J., and Mansi, D.: Musculo Supernumeraris Humero-Radial (Supinador Intermedio). Arch. Soc. Argent. de Anat. Norm. y Path., 4:139–142, 1942.
15. Comtet, J. J., and Chambaud, D.: Paralysie "Spontanée" du Nerf Inter-osseux Postérieur par Lésion Inhabituelle. Deux Observations. Rev. Chir. Orthop., 61:533–541, 1975.
16. Comtet, J.-J., Chambaud, D., and Généty, J.: La Compression de la Branche Postérieure du Nerf Radial. Une Étiologie Méconnue de Certaines Paralysies et de Certaines Épicondylalgies Rebelles. Nouv. Presse Med., 5:1111–1114, 1976.
17. Craig, W. S., and Clark, J. M. P.: Of Peripheral Nerve Palsies in the Newly Born. J. Obstet. Gynecol. Br. Commonw., 65:229–237, 1958.
18. Davies, F., and Laird, M.: The Supinator Muscle and the Deep Radial (Posterior Interosseous) Nerve. Anat. Rec., 101:243–250, 1948.
19. Dharapak, C., and Nimberg, G. A.: Posterior Interosseous Nerve Compression. Report of a Case Caused by Traumatic Aneurysm. Clin. Orthop., 101:225–228, 1974.

20. Duchenne, G. B.: Physiology of Motion. translated and edited by Emanuel B. Kaplan, Philadelphia, W. B. Saunders, 1959, p. 123 and p. 168.
21. Frackelton, W. H., Teasley, J. L., and Tauras, A.: Neuromas in the Hand Treated by Nerve Transposition and Silicone Capping. J. Bone Joint Surg., 53A:813, 1971.
22. Frohse, F., and Frankel, M.: Die Muskeln des Menschlichen Armes. Bardeleben's Handbuch der Anatomie des Menschlichen. Jena, Fisher, 1908.
23. Froment, J.-B.-F.: Traité d'Anatomie Humaine. Paris, Méquignon-Marvis, 1846, p. 494.
24. Gathier, J. C., and Bruyn, G. W.: Peripheral Neuropathies Following the Administration of Heterologous Immune Sera. Psych., Neurol., and Neurochir., 71:351–371, 1968.
25. Goldman, S., Honet, J. C., Sobel, R., and Goldstein, A. S.: Posterior Interosseous-Nerve Palsy in the Absence of Trauma. Arch. Neurol., 21:435–441, 1969.
26. Goldsztaijn, M.: Nieurazowe Uszkodenie Neruv Promieniowlgo Glebokiego. Neurol., Neurochir., Psychiat., Pol., 10:397–400, 1960
27. Grigoresco, D., and Iordanesco, G.: Une Cas Rare de Paralysie Partielle du Nerf Radial. Rev. Neurol., 2:102–104, 1937.
28. Guillain, G., and Courtellemont: L'Action du Muscle Court Supinator dans la Paralysie du Nerf Radial. Presse Med., 13:50–52, 1905.
29. Haines, R. W.: A Revision of the Extensor Muscles of the Forearm in Tetrapods. J. Anat., 73:211–233, 1938–1939.
30. Harburger, A.: Anomalie de Division de la Branche Postérieure du Nerf Radial Extenseur Propre du Medius. Bull. et Mem. Soc. Anat. Paris, 94:236–238, 1924.
31. Hobhouse, N., and Heald, C. B.: A Case of Posterior Interosseous Paralysis. Brit. Med. J., 1:841, April 1936.
32. Hollinshead, W. H.: Anatomy for Surgeons. Vol. 3, The Back and Limbs. 2nd Ed., New York, Hoeber, 1969.
33. Hovelacque, A.: Anatomie des Nerfs Craniels et Rachidiens et du Système Grand Sympathique Chez l'Homme. Vol. 2, Paris, Doin, 1927.
34. Hutton, W. K.: Remarks on the Innervation of the Dorsum Manus with Special Reference to Certain Rare Anomalies. J. Anat. Physiol., 40:326–331, 1906.
35. Jumentié, M. J.: Fausse Griffe Cubitale par Lésion Dissociée du Nerf Radial. Rev. Neurol., 37:756–758, 1921.
36. Kaplan, E. B.: Functional and Surgical Anatomy of the Hand. 2nd Ed., Philadelphia, Lippincott, 1965.
37. Krause, W.: Handbook der Menschlichen Anatomie. Bd. III, Anatomische Varietäten, Hanover, Hahn, 1880.
38. Kruse, F., Jr.: Paralysis of the Dorsal Interosseous Nerve not due to Direct Trauma. A Case Showing Spontaneous Recovery. Neurology, 8:307–308,1958.
39. Lazorthes, G.: Le Système Neuro-vasculaire, Paris, Masson, 1949.
40. LeDouble, A. F.: Traité des Variations du Système Musculaire de l'Homme. Paris, Schleicher, 1897.
41. Lejars, F.: L'Innervation de l'Eminence Thenar. Bull. Soc. Anat. Paris, IV, 5 Series, 433–437, 1890.
42. Levine, J., and Spinner, M.: Neurolysis in the Elderly. Clin. Orthop., 80:13–16, 1971.
43. Learmonth, J. R.: A Variation of the Radial Branch of the Musculo-spiral Nerve. J. Anat., 53:371–372, 1919.
44. Lichter, R., and Jacobsen, T.: Tardy Palsy of the Posterior Interosseous Nerve with Monteggia Fracture. J. Bone Joint Surg., 57A:124–125, 1975.
45. Linell, E. A.: The Distribution of Nerves in the Upper Limb with Reference to Variabilities and Their Clinical Significance. J. Anat., 55:79–112, 1921.
46. Linscheid, R. L.: Injuries to Radial Nerve at Wrist. Arch. Surg., 91:942–946, 1965.
47. von Luschka, H.: Die Anatomie des Menschlichen Körpers. Tübingen, H. Laupp, 1862.
48. Marshall, S. C., and Murray, W. R.: Deep Radial Nerve Palsy Associated with Rheumatoid Arthritis. Clin. Orthop., 103:157–162, 1974.
49. McFarlane, R. M.: Observations on the Functional Anatomy on the Intrinsic Muscles of the Thumb. J. Bone Joint Surg., 44A:1376–1386, 1962.
50. Marie, P., Meige, H., and Patrikios: Paralysie Radiale Dissociée Simulant une Griffe Cubitale. Rev. Neurol., 24:123–124, 1917.
51. Marmor, L., Lawrence, J. F., and Dubois, E.: Posterior Interosseous Nerve Paralysis Due to Rheumatoid Arthritis. J. Bone Joint Surg., 49A:381–383, 1967.
52. Mayer, J. H., and Mayfield, P. H.: Surgery of the Posterior Interosseous Branch of the Radial Nerve. Surg. Gynecol. Obstet., 84:979–982, 1947.
53. Mees, R. A.: Een Verschijnsel Bij Polyneuritis Arsenicosa. Nederl. T. Geneesk, 1:391–396, 1919.

54. Millender, L. H., Nalebuff, E. A., and Holdsworth, D. E.: Posterior Interosseous Nerve Syndrome Secondary to Rheumatoid Synovitis. J. Bone Joint Surg., *55A*:753–757, 1973.
55. Moon, N., and Marmor, L.: Parosteal Lipoma of the Proximal Part of the Radius. J. Bone Joint Surg., *46A*:608–614, 1964.
56. Morris, A. H.: Irreducible Monteggia Lesion with Radial-Nerve Entrapment. J. Bone Joint Surg., *56A*:1744–1746, 1974.
57. Mowell, J. W.: Posterior Interosseous Nerve Injury. Internat. Clin., *2*:188–189, 1921.
58. Mulholland, R. C.: Non-traumatic Progressive Paralysis of the Posterior Interosseous Nerve. J. Bone Joint Surg., *48B*:781–785, 1966.
59. Nancrede, C. B.: Bursae of Elbow and Vicinity. *In* Ashurst, J. Jr. (ed.): The International Encyclopedia of Surgery. New York, William Wood, 1882, p. 711.
60. Nielsen, H. O.: Posterior Interosseous Nerve Paralysis Caused by Fibrous Band Compression at the Supinator Muscle. A Report of Four Cases. Acta Orthop. Scand., *47*:304–307, 1976.
61. Otenasek, F. J.: Progressive Paralysis of the Nervus Dorsalis: Pathological Findings in One Case. Bull. Johns Hopkins Hosp., *81*:163–167, 1947.
62. Paturet, G.: Traité d'Anatomie Humaine. Tome II, Members Supérieur et Inférieur, Paris, Masson, 1951.
63. Phalen, G. S., Kendrick, J. I., and Rodriguez, J. M.: Lipomas of the Upper Extremity. Am. J. Surg., *121*:298–306, 1971.
64. Popelka, S., and Vainio, K.: Entrapment of the Posterior Interosseous Branch of the Radial Nerve in Rheumatoid Arthritis. Acta Orthop. Scand., *45*:370–372, 1974.
65. Rauber, A.: Vater'sche Körper der Bänder und Periostnerven. Inaug. Diss., Münich, 1865.
66. Rauber, A.: Ueber die Nerven der Knochenhaut, und Knochen des Vorderarmes and Unterschenkels. München, C. Fritsch, 1868.
67. Richmond, D. A.: Lipoma Causing a Posterior Interosseous Nerve Lesion. J. Bone Joint Surg., *35B*:83, 1953.
68. Riordan, D. C.: Radial Nerve Paralysis. Orthop. Clin. N. Amer., *5*:283–287, 1974.
69. Roles, N. C., and Maudsley, R. H.: Radial Tunnel Syndrome. Resistant Tennis Elbow as a Nerve Entrapment. J. Bone Joint Surg., *54B*:499–508, 1972.
70. Roussy, G., and Branche, J.: Deux Cas de Paralysies Dissociées de la Branche Postérieure du Radial à Type de Pseudo-Griffe Cubitale. Rev. Neurol., *24*:312–314, 1917.
71. Salsbury, C. R.: The Nerve to the Extensor Carpi Radialis Brevis. Brit. J. Surg., *26*:95–97, 1938.
72. Shäfer, E. A., Symington, J., and Bryce, T. H. (eds.): Quain's Elements of Anatomy. Ed. 11, Vol. 4, Part 2. New York, Longmanns, Green and Co., 1923, pp. 139–140.
73. Sharrard, W. J. W.: Posterior Interosseous Neuritis. J. Bone Joint Surg., *48B*:777–780, 1966.
74. Shevkunenko, V. N.: Atlas of the Peripheral Nervous and Venous Systems. Moscow, Medgiz, 1949.
75. Silverstein, A.: Progressive Paralysis of the Dorsal Interosseous Nerve. Report of a Case. Arch. Neurol. Psychiat., *38*:885–886, 1937.
76. Somerville, E. W.: Pain in the Upper Limb. Proceedings of the British Orthopaedic Association. J. Bone Joint Surg., *45B*:621, 1963.
77. Spinner, M., Freundlich, B. D., and Teicher, J.: Posterior Interosseous Nerve Palsy as a Complication of Monteggia Fracture in Children. Clin. Orthop., *58*:141–145, 1968.
78. Spinner, M.: The Arcade of Frohse and Its Relationship to Posterior Interosseous Nerve Paralysis. J. Bone Joint Surg., *50B*:809–812, 1968.
79. Stein, F., Grabias, S. L., and Deffer, P. A.: Nerve Injuries Complicating Monteggia Lesions. J. Bone Joint Surg., *53A*:1432–1436, 1971.
80. Stookey, B.: Surgical and Mechanical Treatment of Peripheral Nerves. Philadelphia, W. B. Saunders, 1922.
81. Strachan, J. C. H., and Ellis, B. W.: Vulnerability of the Posterior Interosseous Nerve During Radial Head Resection. J. Bone Joint Surg., *53B*:320–323, 1971.
82. Straus, W. L., Jr.: The Phylogeny of the Human Forearm Extensors. Hum. Biol., *13*:23–50, 203–238, 1941.
83. Sunderland, S.: Nerves and Nerve Injuries. Baltimore, Williams & Wilkins, 1968.
84. Sunderland, S.: Traumatic Injuries of Peripheral Nerves. I. Simple Compression Injuries of the Radial Nerve. Brain, *68*:56–72, 1945.
85. Testut, L.: Les Anomalies Musculaire Chez l'Homme. Paris, Masson, 1884.
86. Vaughan-Jackson, O. J.: Rupture of the Extensor Tendons by Attrition at the Inferior Radioulnar Joint. J. Bone Joint Surg., *30B*:528–530, 1948.
87. Voiculescu, V., and Popescu, F.: Non-traumatic Progressive Paralysis of the Deep Branch of the Radial Nerve. Neurologia (Bucur.) *14*:111–115, 1969.
88. Wartenberg, R.: Cheiralgia Paresthetica (Isolierte Neuritis des Ramus Superficialis Nervi Radialis). Zeitschr. f. d. ges. Neurol. Psychiat., *141*:145–155, 1932.

89. Weinberger, L. M.: Non-traumatic Paralysis of the Dorsal Interosseous Nerve. Surg., Gyn., Obst., 69:358–363, 1939.
90. White, W. L., and Hanna, D. C.: Troublesome Lipomata of the Upper Extremity. J. Bone Joint Surg., 44A:1353–1359, 1962.
91. Whitely, W. H., and Alpers, B. J.: Posterior Interosseous Palsy with Spontaneous Neuroma Formation. Arch. Neurol., 1:226–229, 1959.
92. Woltman, H. W., and Kernohan, J. W.: Disease of Peripheral Nerves. In Baker, A. B. (ed.): Clinical Neurology, New York, Hoeber-Harper, 1955, p. 1629.
93. Woltman, H. W., and Learmonth, J. R.: Progressive Paralysis of the Nervus Interosseous Dorsalis. Brain, 57:25–31, 1934.
94. Wood, J.: Variations in Human Myology Observed during the Winter Session of 1867–68 at King's College, London. Proc. Royal Soc. Lond., 16:496, 1868.
95. Wu, K. T., Jordan, F. R., and Eckert, C.: Lipoma, a Cause of Paralysis of Deep Radial (Posterior Interosseous) Nerve. Report of a Case and Review of the Literature. Surgery, 75:790–795, 1974.

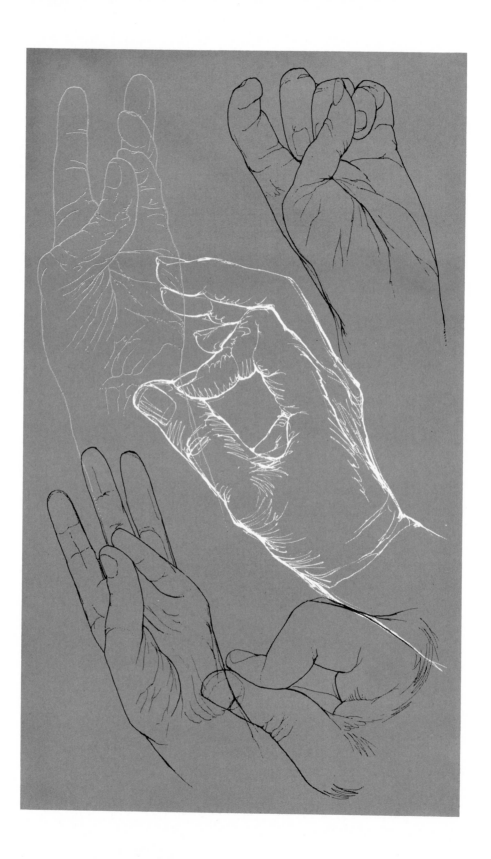

THE MEDIAN NERVE

THE MEDIAN NERVE

ANATOMY

The median nerve, after it has traversed the arm, comes to lie most medial at the level of the distal arm just proximal to the lacertus fibrosus, in close proximity to the brachial artery and the biceps tendon. There is a mnemonic, MAT, which is helpful in remembering the relationship between these structures at the level of the elbow just proximal to the lacertus fibrosus. From the medial epicondyle, M is the median nerve, A is the brachial artery, and T is the biceps tendon. Adjacent to the brachial artery are venae comitantes, two to three of which lie between that artery and the median nerve.

The median nerve in the proximal third of the forearm supplies the flexor pronator group of muscles which arise from the medial epicondyle — the pronator teres, the flexor carpi radialis and the palmaris longus. The proximal portion of the flexor superficialis, which arises from the medial epicondyle and the thickened raphe in the proximal third of the forearm, obtains its motor supply from the motor branches supplying the flexor carpi radialis and the palmaris longus. The motor branches supplying the medial flexor pronator mass usually enter the muscles on their deep or posterior surface.

When the anterior aspect of the forearm in this region is exposed, only the sensory branches—the medial cutaneous nerve of the forearm and the distal portion of the medial cutaneous nerve of the arm (both branches of the medial cord) — are seen superficial to the fascia (Fig. 123). There are no motor nerve branches visible on the anterior aspect of these muscles, but three or four motor branches do arise from the proximal portion of the median nerve in the antecubital region which innervate these muscles—the pronator teres, the flexor carpi radialis, the palmaris longus, and the humeral portion of the flexor digitorum superficialis.

Most usually the pronator teres motor nerve has a common stem with branches to the superficial and deep heads (60 per cent); two separate stems, one going to the superficial and the other to the deep head, may also be found.

The anterior interosseous nerve arises from the median nerve 5 to 8 cm. distal to the level of the lateral epicondyle. During its passage through the forearm it usually innervates three muscles — the flexor pollicis longus, the radial half of the flexor digitorum profundus, and the pronator quadratus. At the end of its course, it supplies sensory fibers to the radiocarpal, intercarpal and carpometacarpal and distal radioulnar joints.

In the region of the superficialis arch, the flexor superficialis is usually innervated by three motor branches from the main median nerve trunk. These branches are located on the deep surface of this muscle.

The palmar cutaneous nerve is the last of the major branches of the median nerve in the forearm. Most commonly, there is one branch arising 5.5 cm. proximal to the radial styloid.

At the wrist, ten structures—the flexor pollicis longus tendon, four flexor digitorum superficialis tendons, four flexor digitorum profundus tendons, and the median nerve—pass from the forearm to the hand through a narrowed, fibro-osseous tunnel, the carpal tunnel. Its walls are the navicular and trapezium on the radial side and the pisiform and hamate on the ulnar side. Its floor is the lunate, capitate, and trapezoid along with their covering ligaments. The roof is the volar carpal ligament. Topographically, the distal volar skin crease of the wrist represents the proximal border of this canal which extends 3 cm. distally from this crease.

The median nerve and its branches supply sympathetic fibers to portions of the vascular tree of the forearm and hand in a segmental fashion. At the elbow, the median nerve delivers a branch to the region of the bifurcation of the brachial artery. It arborizes in the proximal few centimeters of radial and ulnar arteries. The anterior interosseous nerve supplies the anterior interosseous artery with sympathetic fibers, for the most part in the proximal forearm. The sympathetic fibers of the median nerve at the wrist level supply almost completely the superficial palmar arch and, in association with the ulnar nerve, partially supply the deep vascular arch of the hand.

SIGNIFICANT ANATOMICAL VARIATIONS AND CLINICAL APPLICATIONS

Anterior interosseous nerve syndrome.
Gantzer's muscle.
Palmaris profundus.
Flexor carpi radialis brevis.
Pronator syndrome.
Carpal tunnel syndrome.
Martin-Gruber anastomosis.
Accessory motor supply to the flexor superficialis.
Median palmar cutaneous nerve.
Thenar motor branch of the median nerve.
High division of the median nerve.
Riche-Cannieu anastomosis.

Anterior Interosseous Nerve Syndrome

Attention was first focused on the anterior interosseous nerve syndrome by Kiloh and Nevin,[51] in 1952, as an isolated neuritis of this major branch of the median nerve. Tinel,[113] as early as 1918, described this lesion under the title "Dissociated Paralysis of the Median Nerve," briefly noting the findings in two cases. Seyffarth,[96] Bell and Goldner,[5] Thomas,[105] Warren,[116] Fearn and Goodfellow,[27] Stern, Rosner and Blinderman,[111] Farber and Bryan,[26] Sharrard,[98] Mills, Mukherjee and Bassett,[77] and Vichare[114] have all made contributions to the understanding of the subject. Recently, Assmus, Homer, and Martin,[2] Benini and Tedeschi,[6] Bucher,[10] De Vecchis,[21] Finelli,[29] Gardner-Thorpe,[35] Huffmann and Leven,[44] Krag,[54] Lake,[56] Luppino, Celli, and Montelone,[64] Maeda et al.,[65] Nakano, Lundergan and Okihiro,[80] O'Brien and Upton,[81] Schmidt and Eiken,[94] Smith and Herbst,[99] and Passerini and Vall[86] have added to the knowledge. The earlier related studies of Borchardt and Wjasmenski,[7] Ranschburg,[90] Wilson,[98] Parsonage and Turner,[85] and subsequent reports of Furusawa et al.[32] and Matsuzaki et al.[73] are significant contributions to the subject.

Personal clinical and anatomical studies[101, 102] indicate that several factors may play a part in the production of paralysis of an anterior interosseous nerve. Near its site of origin this motor branch is vulnerable to injury or compression by the following means:

1. A tendinous origin of the deep head of the pronator teres (Fig. 69).

2. A tendinous origin of the flexor superficialis to the long finger.

3. A thrombosis of crossing ulnar collateral vessels (Fig. 69B).

4. An accessory muscle and tendon from the flexor superficialis to the flexor pollicis longus.

5. An accessory head of the flexor pollicis longus (Gantzer's muscle) (Fig. 70).

6. An aberrant radial artery.

7. A tendinous origin of variant muscles, the palmaris profundus or flexor carpi radialis brevis (Fig. 89A and B).

8. An enlarged bicipital bursa encroaching on the median nerve near the region of the origin of the anterior interosseous nerve.

TYPES OF CLINICAL PRESENTATIONS OF ANTERIOR INTEROSSEOUS NERVE PARALYSIS.   There are several ways in which an anterior interosseous nerve paralysis may manifest itself. The clinical pattern depends to the greatest extent on whether the neural lesion is complete or partial. In addition, the clinical presentation can be affected by specific anatomical variations that may exist in a particular limb. Thus, the clinical pattern may differ even with complete lesions.

The typical anterior interosseous nerve syndrome presents usually

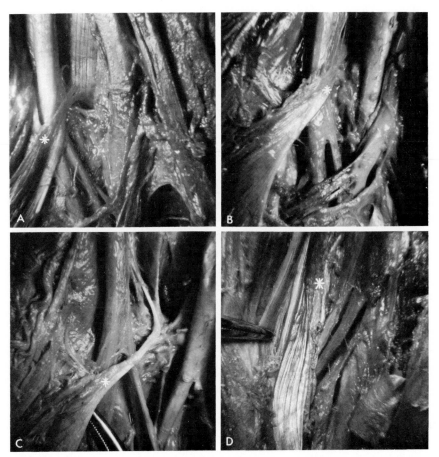

Figure 69.   Left anatomical specimens. The variations of tendinous origin of the deep head of the pronator teres (*) are demonstrated. *A*, A tendinous loop is formed about the median nerve at the level of the takeoff of the anterior interosseous branch. *B*, In addition to the tendinous origin of the deep head of the pronator teres, the crossing ulnar collateral vessels are noted more distal. *C*, The thinnest tendinous origin noted. *D*, The broadest. The tendinous origin is noted across the hila of the anterior interosseous nerve as it arises from the main median nerve trunk.

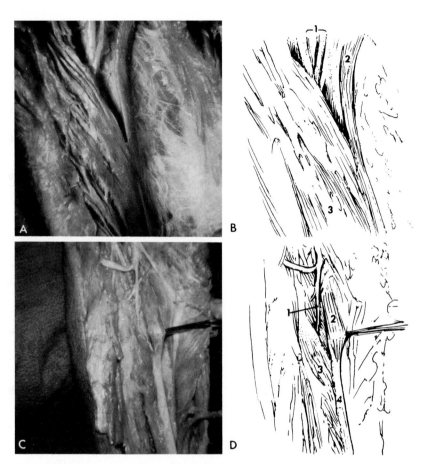

Figure 70.   Right anatomical specimens. *A*, Demonstrates the usual size of Gantzer's muscle (2), an accessory head of the flexor pollicis longus (3) and its relationship to the anterior interosseous nerve (1). *C*, The largest Gantzer's muscle seen in this anatomical study attaching to the flexor pollicis longus tendon (4).

with a history of pain in the proximal forearm of several hours' duration. Pain subsides only to be followed by a paresis or total paralysis of the flexor pollicis longus and the flexor profundus of the index finger and the long finger. The pronator quadratus is usually paralyzed. The pronator teres, however, is unaffected.

The partial interosseous nerve lesion presents with an isolated inability to flex the terminal phalanx of the thumb, index, long or ring finger. Conceivably, the pronator quadratus alone can be paralyzed, but the pathological process may go unrecognized clinically because of the uninvolved pronator teres.

The hand that presents with an anterior interosseous paralysis has a typical appearance with a characteristic disturbance of pinch (Fig. 71*A*). The clinical picture of an anterior interosseous nerve paralysis is as

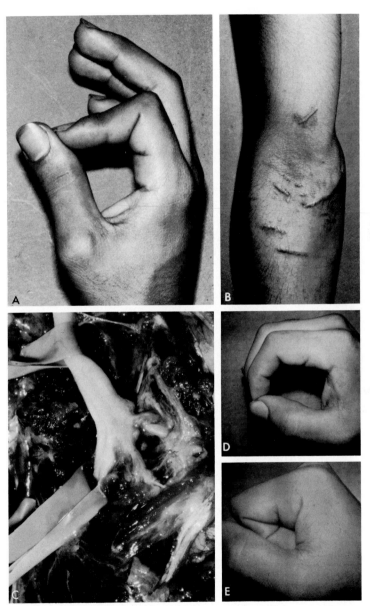

Figure 71.   *A*, The right hand has an anterior interosseous nerve paralysis. The pinch attitude of this hand is characteristic of this paralysis. *B*, Note the multiple stab wounds of the right forearm. *C*, The neuroma involves only a portion of the median nerve. *D*, Following tendon transfers, the pinch attitude has returned to normal. *E*, Flexion of the terminal phalanx of the thumb and index finger is restored.

constant as that presented by other well-known peripheral nerve injuries.

A presumptive diagnosis of an anterior interosseous nerve paralysis
can be made from the attitude of the thumb and index finger during
pinch. Normally, there are varying degrees of flexion of all joints of the
thumb and index finger. With an anterior interosseous nerve paralysis,
the index finger shows extension of the distal interphalangeal joint and
increased flexion of the proximal interphalangeal joint. The involved
thumb reveals increased flexion of the metacarpophalangeal joint and
hyperextension of the interphalangeal joint. In addition, the pulp contact
between the thumb and index finger is abnormal, the area of contact of
the pulp of the thumb with the index finger being more proximal than
normal (Fig. 71A).

Confirmatory findings of an anterior interosseous nerve paralysis
include a lack of function of the long flexors of the thumb and index and
long fingers as well as lack of function of the pronator quadratus of the
forearm. There is no sensory abnormality or involvement of other muscles
supplied by the main median nerve trunk.

With the common distribution of the median nerve, the superficial
flexors, lumbricals, thenar muscles, and the deep flexors to the ring and
little fingers are normal. In the extreme "all median hand," the anterior
interosseous nerve supplies all of the flexor profundus muscles. Accordingly, in this and the other variants of the median nerve the attitude of
the thumb and index finger in the pinch position would be the same as
described, but there would be weakness or paralysis of some or all of the
components of the flexor digitorum profundus. Conversely, when the
ulnar nerve innervates more of the profundi, the long finger profundus
is unaffected or is only partially paralyzed by loss of function of the
anterior interosseous nerve. In this case, the involved hand would have
the same pinch attitude as described, but the flexor profundus of the
long finger would be either weak or normal (Fig. 72A and B).

Sunderland[107] has observed that "the portion of the flexor digitorum
profundus serving the index finger is the only part of this muscle that is
exclusively and constantly supplied by the median nerve." Theoretically,
if the ulnar nerve did supply the entire flexor profundus group of muscles, then a lesion of the anterior interosseous nerve would be manifested
only by lack of flexion of the interphalangeal joint of the thumb and
paralysis of the pronator quadratus. One such rare case was reported by
Sunderland.[109]

In testing for function of the pronator quadratus, one must eliminate the rotary action of the pronator teres on the forearm by fully
flexing the elbow. Since the pronator teres usually has two heads, the
humeral head can be made ineffective by flexing the elbow so that only
about 25 per cent of the muscle's pronatory strength from the ulnar head

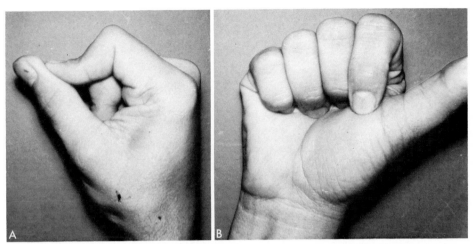

Figure 72.   *A*, A typical pinch attitude of anterior interosseous nerve paralysis in the right hand. The patient opposes his thumb well. *B*, Only the terminal phalanx of the index finger and thumb cannot flex. In this patient the flexor digitorum profundus to the long finger is innervated by the ulnar nerve.

remains. In this position if there is a paralysis of the pronator quadratus there would be very weak resistance to forced supination of the forearm, whereas if the pronator quadratus is not paralyzed, resistance to supination will be normal when the elbow is flexed or extended. When the pronator teres has no ulnar head (a variation found in 9 per cent of limbs) there will be at most only a trace of active pronation in the presence of an anterior interosseous nerve paralysis when the elbow is fully flexed. The clinical evaluation of the function of the pronator quadratus can be corroborated by direct electrical stimulation of the muscle.

Bilateral anterior interosseous nerve paralysis can occur (Fig. 73*A* and *B*).

Variations.   There are additional variations that can occur in an anterior interosseous nerve syndrome. The Martin-Gruber type of communication between the median and ulnar nerves occurs in 15 per cent of limbs.[112] Half of these communications have been reported to arise from the anterior interosseous nerve (Fig. 74). This communication between the median and ulnar nerve is of significance because the anastomosing fibers carry the motor innervation of several of the intrinsic muscles of the hand. Mannerfelt[68] demonstrated that these crossing fibers may innervate the first dorsal interosseous, the adductor pollicis and probably the abductor digiti quinti. Morrison and I[79] confirmed Mannerfelt's observations by electrical methods.

In addition to the intrinsic muscles previously mentioned, the second and third dorsal interosseous muscles were also found to be supplied by

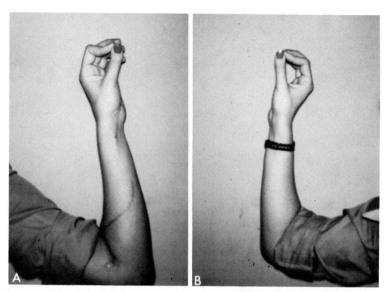

Figure 73.   *A*, A 26-year-old female teacher developed an anterior interosseous nerve paralysis of her left forearm while playing tennis. While recuperating from surgery and while swimming, she developed a similar paralysis in the opposite forearm (*B*). Note the typical pinch attitude of an anterior interosseous nerve paralysis of the right forearm.

these crossing fibers in some limbs. Thus, a patient with a full-blown anterior interosseous nerve paralysis not only may have the usual dysfunction of the deep flexors of the thumb, index fingers and long finger, and the pronator quadratus, but may also have paralysis of some intrinsic muscles of the hand. Such a communication is a not too infrequent anatomical variation.

Furthermore, Sunderland has noted that the anterior interosseous nerve in six of 20 upper limb specimens supplied a branch to the flexor superficialis, an incidence of 30 per cent. The specimens had, in addition, separate branches to the flexor superficialis from the main median nerve trunk, so that it is possible in a full-blown anterior interosseous nerve palsy to have impairment not only of the long flexor muscle of the thumb and the deep flexor muscles of the index and long fingers but also of some of the intrinsics and variable weakness of the flexor superficialis muscles.

In another variation of the syndrome, an isolated paralysis of the flexor pollicis longus can occur and must be differentiated from a rupture of that muscle or its tendon. Some of the intrinsic muscles of the hand, especially the first dorsal interosseous, adductor pollicis, abductor digiti quinti, and the second and third dorsal interossei, may show gross paralysis or partial electrical denervation in an anterior interosseous nerve syndrome. The finding of intrinsic muscle involvement with paral-

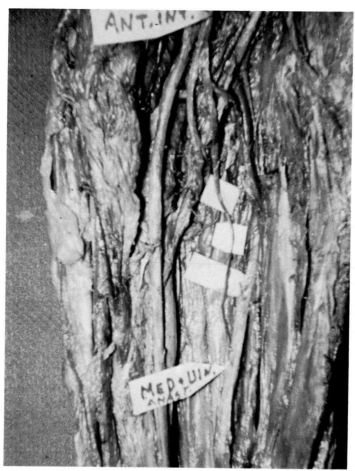

Figure 74.   Right forearm specimen. Note the Martin-Gruber type communication between the median and ulnar nerves through a branch of the anterior interosseous nerve. The humeral origin of the flexor superficialis has been detached to expose the details of the anastomosis. (Courtesy of Dr. Emanual B. Kaplan.)

ysis of the long flexors of the thumb and the index finger and long fingers and the pronator quadratus is not inconsistent with a diagnosis of injury to the anterior interosseous nerve in the proximal portion of the forearm. In addition, a minimal paresis of the flexor superficialis muscles is also not inconsistent with this diagnosis. This reflects Sunderland's observation that at times the flexor superficialis may have some innervation from the anterior interosseous nerve.

DIFFERENTIAL DIAGNOSIS.   In differential diagnosis of a hand presenting with a loss of flexion of the thumb and the distal phalanx of the index finger (the anterior interosseous nerve syndrome), one must consider the *neuritis* described by Parsonage and Turner[85] wherein absence of flexion of the distal phalanx of the thumb is associated with variable weakness of the scapular muscles. The presence of more proximal limb muscle involvement gives the clue to this syndrome, thus distinguishing it from a localized entrapment in the forearm.

In *rheumatoid disease* when there are attritional changes of the flexor tendons on the radial side of the carpal tunnel associated with local subluxation of the midcarpal joint with prominence of the volarly sub-luxed carpal bone, rupture of the flexor pollicis longus and the flexor profundus of the index finger is possible. The pinch attitude of this rheumatoid arthritic hand would be similar to that of the anterior in-terosseous nerve syndrome.

We have seen a *congenital absence* of the deep flexors of the hand with congenital absence of the flexor pollicis longus and all flexor digitorum profundus muscles. Pinch in this hand gave a similar attitude and had to be distinguished from that seen in the patient with an anterior interos-seous nerve syndrome (Fig. 75). A history that reveals that the patient was born with the absence of muscles in the hand and, often, in the legs, coupled with electrical evaluation, helps confirm the diagnosis of this congenital condition.

James[45] reported a case of rupture of flexor tendons secondary to *Kienböck's disease.* The hand afflicted with rupture of the flexor pollicis longus and flexor profundus of the index finger produces a similar pathological pinch position. However, the pronator quadratus would function normally and would have a normal EMG pattern. This helps confirm the diagnosis of tendon rupture. Furthermore, wrist movement would be decreased in this instance because of the carpal bone pathology.

A unique partial lesion of the median nerve or the lateral root of the median nerve arising from the lateral cord in the axilla can mimic an anterior interosseous nerve paralysis.[103] An unusual type of mechanism in some cases of spontaneous infraclavicular brachial plexus neuritis may be due to perforation of these specific terminal components of the plexus by anomalous branches of the axillary vessels. With repeated abduction of the shoulder, a local, mechanically induced neuropathy may be pro-duced. This is exemplified by the following case.

A 25-year-old white female noted severe pain in the right shoulder for 10 days and then sudden inability to flex the terminal phalanx of her thumb. There was no sensory or other motor weakness. On physical examination maximum tenderness was observed at the level of the coracoid process. When the neurovascular bundle was percussed, pain was elicited from the coracoid process to the upper half of the arm (Fig. 76A). There was complete paralysis of the flexor pollicis longus, but no other motor loss was noted (Fig. 76B). There was no sensory abnormality in either hand or upper extremity. Neuro-logical examination was otherwise normal. There was no change in the pulse of either arm with change of position of the arm, even with full abduction and extension of the shoulder. The Adson test was negative. Electromyographic studies revealed fibrillations only in the flexor pollicis longus muscle in the right forearm. There was no conduction disturbance in the main peripheral nerves of the upper extremities.

Text continued on page 174

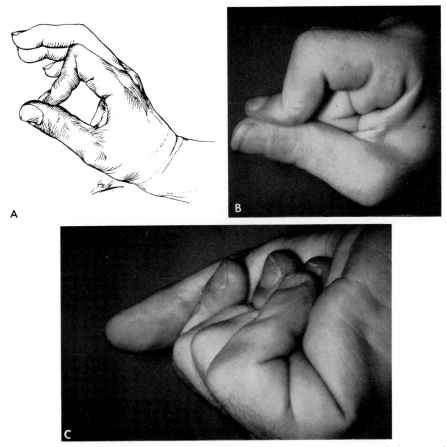

Figure 75.   *A,* Note the characteristic pinch attitude seen in paralysis of the anterior interosseous nerve. *B,* The right hand in the pinch position in a patient with congenital absence of the flexor pollicis longus and flexor profundi to all the fingers (*C*). There is normal opposition of the thumb.

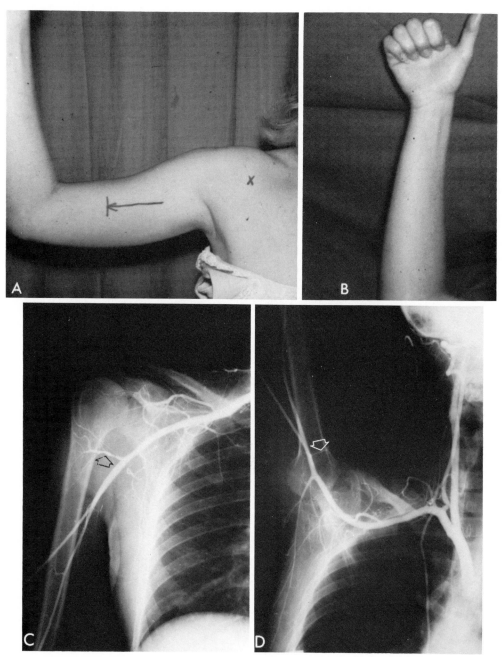

Figure 76.   *A*, Pain in the patient's right shoulder was maximum just distal to the coracoid process (X). There was percussion tenderness along the neurovascular bundle of
the proximal segment of the arm. *B*, She was unable to flex the terminal phalanx of the
thumb. Her fingers flexed fully. *C*, Subclavian arteriography performed with the arm at
the side revealed a segmental narrowing and irregular filling of the posterior humeral
circumflex artery (arrow). *D*, The arteriography was repeated with the arm abducted.
The posterior humeral circumflex artery did not fill. The anterior circumflex artery
(arrow) is noted.

Illustration continued on opposite page

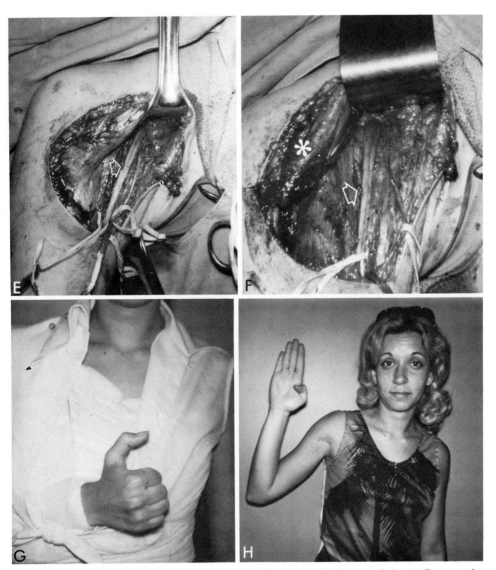

Figure 76 *Continued.* *E*, At operation the ligated posterior humeral circumflex vessels (arrow) had penetrated the median nerve, splitting it into two parts. *F*, The pectoralis major (asterisk) was retracted after the distal half of its tendon was divided. The median nerve was explored more proximally to the level of the coracoid process. No other pathology was found. *G*, By the fourth postoperative day, in the Velpeau dressing, weak flexion of the terminal phalanx of the thumb was noted. *H*, Complete flexion of the distal phalanx of the thumb, and normal strength of the flexor pollicis longus, was found four months after surgery.

Subclavian arteriography was performed with the right arm at the side, and at 90 degrees abduction.

Roentgenographic studies revealed an abnormality of the posterior humeral circumflex artery. With the arm at the side, this vessel was noted to be wavy and segmentally narrowed (Fig. 76C). With the arm abducted and subclavian arteriography repeated, this vessel was completely cut off and did not fill (Fig. 76D).

Surgical exploration of the infraclavicular portion of the brachial plexus was performed. Through a broad-based, continuous, zig-zag surgical incision, which avoided crossing the anterior axillary fold, the median nerve and the brachial artery and vein were identified and traced proximally. The posterior humeral circumflex vein and artery were found to penetrate the median nerve. These vessels had split the proximal portion of the median nerve and the lateral root of the median nerve into two parts (Fig. 76E). These anomalous perforating major vessels were ligated. The median nerve and its neural roots were explored up to the level of the coracoid process. No other pathology was found proximal to the level of the vascular perforation (Fig. 76F).

The intense preoperative pain in the right shoulder disappeared immediately following surgery. Furthermore, a trace of motion in the flexor pollicis longus was noted during the first few postoperative days (Fig. 76G). The patient had progressive improvement in the function of her right thumb, so much so that by the end of the fourth postoperative month she had full strength and full range of excursion of the flexor pollicis longus (Fig. 76H).

This case must be differentiated from one with a classic anterior interosseous nerve syndrome in which the flexor pollicis longus, as well as the flexor profundus to both the index and long fingers, and the pronator quadratus are paralyzed. On occasion, a partial anterior interosseous nerve paralysis occurs in which only the flexor pollicis longus is paralyzed. The location of pain can be helpful in establishing the proper diagnosis. The patient had severe pain in the region of the shoulder with a positive Tinel sign. When pain does occur in an anterior interosseous nerve paralysis, the pain is usually in the proximal forearm.

Miller,[76] in a study of 480 human extremities, reported an 8 per cent aberrant relationship between the axillary artery and the brachial plexus. A variant posterior humeral circumflex artery, or a common stem for the posterior and anterior humeral circumflex vessels, can penetrate the median nerve just distal to its formation, splitting it in two. In addition, these vessels can in a similar manner penetrate the lateral root of the median nerve of the lateral cord (Fig. 77A). A variant subscapular artery can also penetrate the median nerve in this region (Fig. 77B).

It is suggested that some of the idiopathic cases of brachial plexus neuritis may be due to a neural compression lesion.[103] The compression is caused by anomalous perforation of the components of the infraclavicular portion of the brachial plexus or their most proximal peripheral nerves by large arterial or venous branches of the axillary vessels. When the shoulder is abducted, these perforating vascular branches can tether the nerve. As the abduction motion is repeated, isolated episodes of brachial plexus neuritis can occur. If the condition is not treated, repeated or recurrent episodes of brachial plexus neuritis with possible paralysis may be experienced.

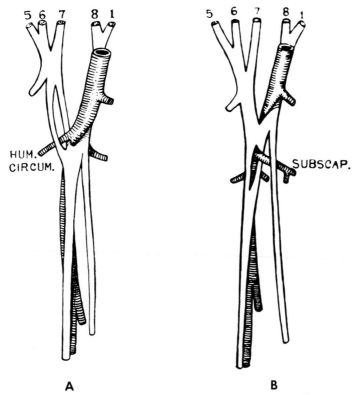

Figure 77.   *A*, Anomalous perforation of the lateral root of the median nerve by the posterior humeral circumflex artery. The median nerve also can be penetrated by this vessel. *B*, Perforation of the median nerve by the subscapular artery has also been described. (From Miller, R. A.: Observations upon the Arrangement of the Axillary Artery and the Brachial Plexus. Am. J. Anat., *64*:161, 1939.)

It is also recommended that subclavian arteriography and venography with the arm in abduction and at the side be included, in addition to the routine clinical examinations, laboratory testing, myelography and electrodiagnostic measures, in evaluating a presumptive diagnosis of brachial plexus neuritis.

In other instances, penetration of the median nerve in the axilla by major anomalous vascular branches has presented with paralysis of the flexor pollicis longus, pronator quadratus and pronator teres in one case, and with paralysis of the flexor pollicis longus, pronator quadratus, pronator teres, flexor carpi radialis and palmaris longus in another. There was no sensory abnormality in the hand, and the other median innervated muscles in the forearm and hand functioned normally. Following release of the median nerve by ligation of the offending vessel, the axillary pain subsided in the immediate postoperative period. Neural recovery followed in the expected manner observed with a combined neurapractic and axonotmetic lesion.

Lastly, in differential diagnosis, there is the possibility of a *lesion of the medial root* of the median nerve, as indicated in the following case. An elderly white male was first seen 6 weeks after sustaining an anterior dislocation of the shoulder with inability to flex the terminal phalanx of the thumb. Examination revealed paralysis of the flexor profundus of the index finger and paresis of the flexor profundus of the long finger, in addition to paralysis of the thenar muscles. The flexor carpi radialis and the pronator teres were normal in strength. Since these latter two muscles are innervated by funiculi that traverse the lateral root of the median nerve, they were spared. Sensory examination was normal. Woltman[120] has described paralysis of the flexor pollicis longus associated with a lesion of the medial root of the median nerve.

Sunderland notes that the anterior interosseous funiculi pass through both the *medial* and *lateral* roots of the median nerve.

Isolated paralysis of the flexor pollicis longus can occur and has been seen in association with an enlarged bicipital bursa *compressing* the anterior interosseous nerve. It has also been observed as a variant of the anterior interosseous nerve syndrome where the compressing structures may be the tendinous origin of the flexor superficialis of the long finger and thrombosed collateral vessels of the anterior interosseous artery. The isolated paralysis must be differentiated from a traumatic rupture of the flexor pollicis longus (Fig. 78). Electromyographic studies can help distinguish the two. Fibrillations of the flexor pollicis longus muscle, and often of the pronator quadratus, support the diagnosis of denervation.

CAUSES.   I have seen 35 cases of anterior interosseous nerve syndromes: twelve were due to entrapment structures, six were caused by perforating wounds, seven resulted from supracondylar fractures in children, six stemmed from open reduction of fractures of the radius midshaft and four were due to compression of both the median nerve and anterior interosseous nerves.

Entrapment.   A typical example of entrapment of the anterior interosseous nerve secondary to tendinitis of the deep head of the pronator teres was found in a 13-year-old boy who was first seen on April 1, 1968. Two months earlier he had lifted a heavy bundle of papers on his newspaper route. He noted pain in his left forearm, and shortly thereafter was unable to bend the thumb. His left index finger was noted to be weak.

When he was seen initially there was no sensory abnormality, the pain had disappeared and a Tinel sign was absent. The flexor pollicis longus and the pronator quadratus did not function. The flexor profundus of the index finger showed a trace of action, while the flexor profundus muscles to the long, ring and little fingers were normal. The flexor superficialis muscle and all the intrinsics of the hand were of normal strength.

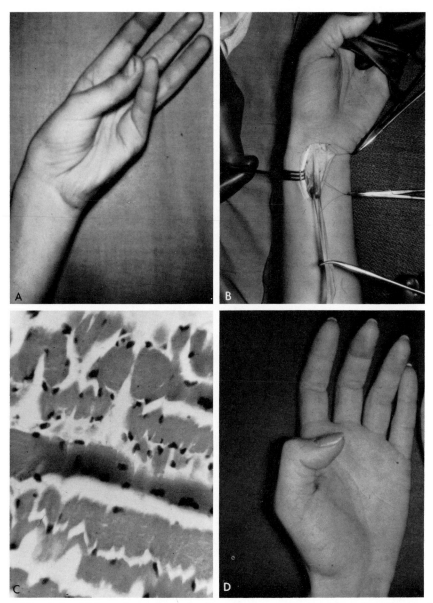

Figure 78.   After lifting a heavy bag of coins, the patient was unable to flex the terminal phalanx of the left thumb. *B*, There is no rupture of the flexor pollicis longus. The terminal phalanx flexes on traction of the musculotendinous junction of this muscle. *C*, Biopsy specimen of the flexor pollicis longus taken at the time of the transfer of the flexor superficialis of the ring finger to the flexor pollicis longus tendon. The increase in the number of nuclei about the muscle fibers is indicative of denervation (hematoxylin and eosin, × 1000). *D*, Postoperative flexion of the terminal phalanx of the thumb is complete.

Electromyography revealed fibrillations of the pronator quadratus and the flexor pollicis longus. Exploration of the median nerve was performed on April 29, 1968. The median nerve was identified proximal to the lacertus fibrosis and traced through the pronator teres, where it passed between the two heads. Adhesions were seen about the median nerve and the deep head of the pronator teres. When these were cleared a

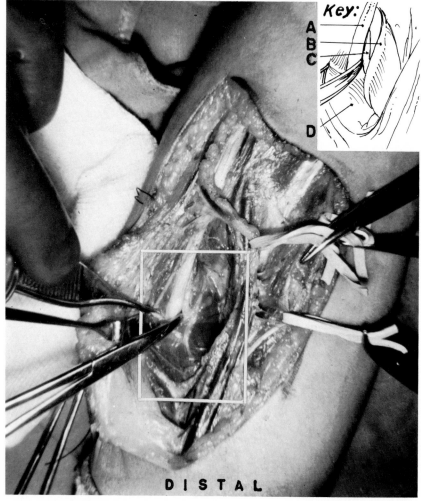

Figure 79.   Left forearm. The median nerve is exposed proximal to the lacertus fibrosus and is traced to its passage through both heads of the pronator teres. Adhesions about the muscle have been cleared. The anterior interosseous nerve is in direct contact with the deep tendinous head of the pronator teres. The hemostat is at the axilla of the anterior interosseous nerve. (Key: *A*, median nerve; *B*, tendinous origin of deep head of pronator teres; *C*, anterior interosseous nerve; *D*, superficial head of pronator teres.)

distinct tendinous origin of the deep head of the pronator teres was found (Fig. 79). After this deep tendinous origin was released and an internal neurolysis of the interosseous nerve was performed with the injection of normal saline, the vessels on the surface of the median nerve filled with blood and became visible. The limb was immobilized in a cast for 3 weeks postoperatively. Within a few days, function returned to the flexor profundus of the index finger. By 3 weeks, contraction of the flexor pollicis longus was first evident. By the sixth postoperative week, there was normal power in the flexor pollicis longus, flexor profundus of the index finger and the pronator quadratus. Biopsy of the specimen of the tendon of the deep head of the pronator teres revealed nonspecific tendinitis.

The recovery pattern of the patient after neurolysis suggests that the nerve lesion was a mixed neurapraxia and axonotmesis. The prompt return of full function in the flexor profundus to the index finger is indicative of neurapraxia. The fibrillations and delayed recovery in the flexor pollicis longus and the pronator quadratus suggest axonotmesis with wallerian degeneration.

That the tendinous origin of the deep head of the pronator teres is the most frequent etiological anatomical factor in the production of this paralysis is illustrated by typical operative findings (Fig. 80*A* and *B*).

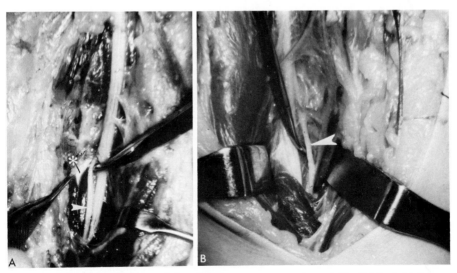

Figure 80. *A*, The tendinous origin of the pronator teres (asterisk) of this right forearm demonstrates at operation its relationship to the anterior interosseous nerve. In this region the anterior interosseous nerve is devoid of vascular markings (arrow). *B*, Note similar lack of vascular markings of the anterior interosseous nerve (arrow) in this left forearm. The tendinous origin of the deep head of the pronator teres has been released.

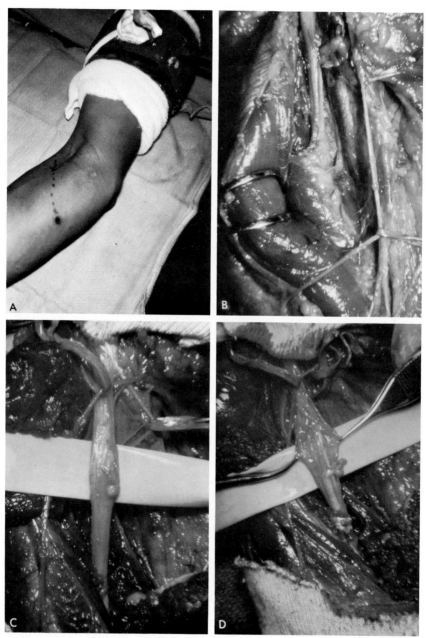

Figure 81.   Left arm. *A*, The course of the bullet is noted commencing approximately at the medial epicondylar region and traversing obliquely to the radial aspect of the forearm. *B*, Adhesions and scarring are seen about the median nerve in the region of the two heads of the pronator. *C*, The adhesions have been cleared. Note the small neuroma of the posterior lateral portion of the median nerve. *D*, The median nerve has been opened. Two fasciculi were found disrupted. The epineurium is held by the forceps.

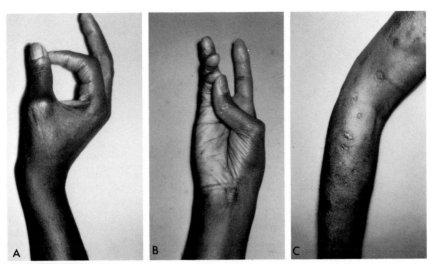

Figure 82.   An anterior interosseous nerve paralysis in the right upper limb of a drug addict.

Perforating Wounds.   We have seen cases of interosseous nerve paralysis as a result of stab wounds of the proximal forearm (Fig. 71), bullet wounds (Fig. 81) and as a result of the injections by drug addicts (Fig. 82). Sunderland[108] has demonstrated that the interosseous nerve becomes a separate bundle approximately 2.5 cm. proximal to its departure from the main trunk of the median nerve at a point 224 to 234 mm. proximal to the radial styloid process (Fig. 83). Thus the anterior interosseous branch of the median nerve or the fascicular component of the median nerve can sustain isolated injury. The significance of this was clearly documented clinically in the following case.

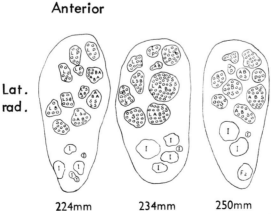

Figure 83.   Internal topography of the median nerve at the involved level. The I fibers are those of the anterior interosseous nerve; F_2 fibers are those of the flexor superficialis. (From Sidney Sunderland: The Intraneural Topography of the Radial, Median, and Ulnar Nerves. Brain, *68*:243–299, 1945.)

A 45-year-old male was stabbed many times through his abdomen, chest and left elbow with a stiletto-type knife. Clinically the patient had sustained a combined radial and anterior interosseous nerve paralysis (Fig. 84A–D). This was confirmed by surgical exploration (Fig. 84E–G). The multiple nerve injuries were not repaired until the seventh day because concomitant lung and liver perforations took priority. Return of function

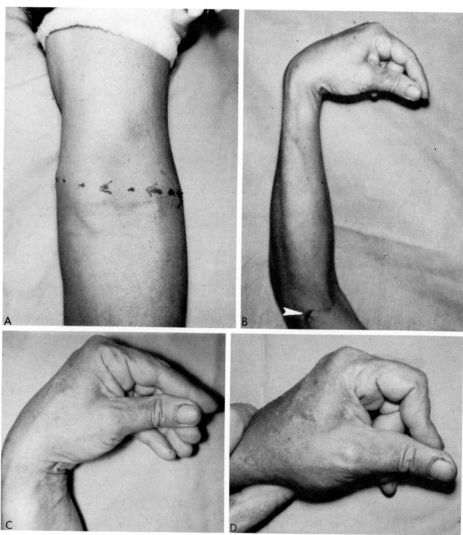

Figure 84.   *A*, The course of the thin knife that entered the lateral side of the left elbow at the antecubital crease and passed through the soft tissues anterior to the elbow joint is noted. *B*, The patient was unable to extend his wrist and fingers, typical of a complete high radial nerve paralysis. Note the knife entrance wound (arrow). *C*, When he pinched his thumb and index finger, this pinch attitude was noted. His wrist was in a flexed position. *D*, When his wrist was supported in a neutral position the typical pinch attitude of an anterior interosseous nerve paralysis was observed.

Illustration continued on opposite page

was excellent. He returned to his usual employment as a waiter in 3 months. Complete function was restored to the radial nerve and anterior interosseous funicular component of the median nerve within 6 months. It is interesting to note, as demonstrated by this case, that the classic pinch attitude seen in anterior interosseous nerve paralysis can be masked by other, coincidental, nerve paralysis.

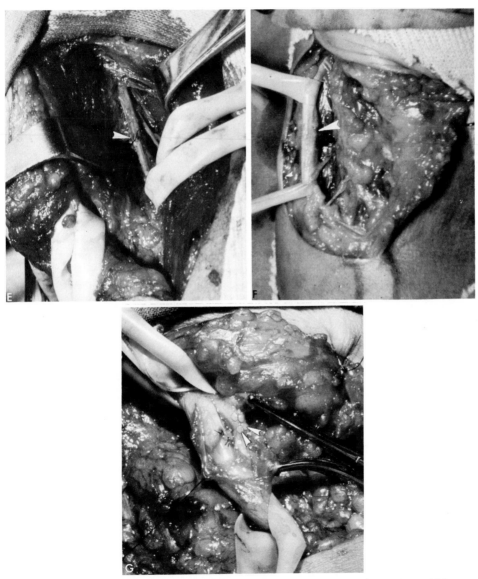

Figure 84 *Continued.* *E*, In addition to a complete radial nerve laceration which was repaired (arrow), a partial laceration of the posterior aspect of the median nerve (arrow) was demonstrated through a separate incision (*F*). *G*, Four anterior interosseous funiculi were found to have been lacerated. Two are repaired with 9–0 nylon. The other two funiculi (arrows) were repaired after this photograph was taken.

Another case commenced 10 years after a deep puncture wound of the forearm, initially causing no difficulty. Others immediately followed the initial injury.[102]

Fracture Complications

Radial fractures.   The anterior interosseous nerve and its branches are vulnerable to injury in open reduction of fractures of the midshaft of the radius and in the muscle slide procedure. Page,[83] in his original description of the procedure, drew attention to this.

The motor branch of the flexor pollicis longus can be injured during open reduction of fractures of the mid-third of the radius if the dissection is extraperiosteal. I have treated two such patients who had normal flexion of the profundus muscles to the remaining digits and normal pronator quadratus action, clinically and electrically, but were unable to flex the interphalangeal joint of the thumb. Transfer of the flexor superficialis of the ring finger to the flexor pollicis longus tendon at the proper tension yielded return of full flexion of the thumb.

Supracondylar fractures.   With regard to the probable mechanism of anterior interosseous nerve paralysis when seen as a complication of supracondylar fractures of the humerus in children, it is my opinion that in six cases that I have seen, along with the four cases noted by Lipscomb and Burleson[62] and those mentioned by Fahey,[25] the injury may have been due to traction on the anterior interosseous nerve in the proximal portion of the forearm rather than to a contusion of the posterior aspect of the median nerve at the level of the supracondylar fracture.[101] The specificity of the motor loss without sensory loss makes partial median nerve injury secondary to contusion unlikely.

As further evidence of traction of the anterior interosseous nerve as a cause for its paralysis Sunderland's cross-sectional map of the median nerve in the supracondylar region (Fig. 85C) reveals that direct posterior injury to the median nerve would injure the fibers innervating the pronator teres and the flexor superficialis in addition to the anterior interosseous nerve component. Furthermore, sensory fibers to the forearm are situated immediately anterior to the fibers of the anterior interosseous nerve. Blunt trauma to the posterior aspect of the median nerve sufficient to produce total paralysis of these muscles would not completely spare the sensory fibers in the immediate proximity of these motor fibers. The possibility that the nerve injury may have been caused by an impending Volkmann's ischemia is refuted by the absence of pain on passive extension of the flexed finger and by absence of other ischemic signs (median nerve sensory loss, loss of deep capillary circulation, pulselessness, cyanosis and subsequent paralysis).

Since the clinical pattern in our patients was one of specific motor loss involving only the muscles innervated by the anterior interosseous nerve without involvement of the main median nerve trunk, I believe that the

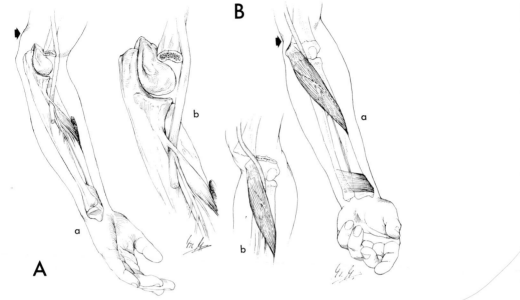

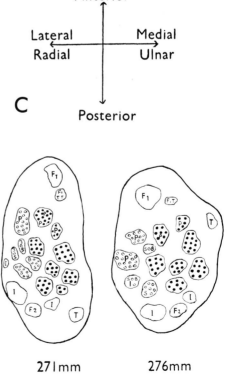

Figure 85. *A*, Lateral view depicts the probable mechanism for production of an anterior interosseous nerve paralysis associated with a supracondylar fracture of the humerus. The fracture and displacement of the supracondylar fragment of the humerus posteriorly tenses the median nerve between the proximal shaft and the fibrous arch of the deep head of the pronator teres. The anterior interosseous nerve arising from the radial aspect of the median nerve is compressed at the level of the fibrous arch in the proximal third of the forearm. b, Spot view of the involved area. *B*, Anteroposterior view. a, The undisplaced anatomical relationship of the median nerve to the pronator teres. The anterior interosseous nerve usually arises at the level of the deep head of the pronator teres. b, The displacement of the fracture fragments and its relationship to the median nerve. *C*, Cross section of the median nerve at the supracondylar level: 271 mm. is immediately proximal to the humeral condyles. I, Anterior interosseous fibers; F_1, proximal common flexor fibers; F_2, distal common flexor fibers; T, pronator teres; S, flexor digitorum superficialis; P, palmar cutaneous fibers; solid dots, combined terminal and flexor digitorum superficialis fibers; circles, combined muscle and cutaneous fibers from the thumb and the first interspace. (From Sunderland, S.: The Intraneural Topography of the Radial, Median and Ulnar Nerves. Brain, *68*:243–299, 1945.)

mechanism for producing the paralysis in these instances is traction. A distal point of fixation of the anterior interosseous nerve and posterior displacement of the distal fragment are prerequisites for the nerve injury. In patients in whom the median nerve slips between the fracture fragments, rather than being completely anterior with the proximal fragment, isolated involvement of the anterior interosseous nerve was not noted.

Experiments were performed on cadaver limbs with the deep tendinous head of the pronator teres intact and the lacertus fibrosus resutured, and an oteotomy of the humerus in the supracondylar region was produced. When the distal fragment was brought anteriorly, laterally or medially there was no increased compression on the anterior interosseous nerve. With posterior displacement of the distal fragment of the humerus, there was definite increased compression at the level of the takeoff of the anterior interosseous nerve from the median nerve trunk in the region of the deep tendinous origin of the pronator teres (Fig. 85A and B). Seven of the 30 limbs that were dissected presented an arch of tough fibrous tissue. Anatomical structures that might participate in the pathological mechanism are as follows: (1) an accessory head of the flexor pollicis longus (Gantzer's muscle); (2) thrombosed ulnar collateral vessels; (3) an accessory muscle from the flexor superficialis to the flexor pollicis longus; (4) the deep tendinous head of the pronator teres; and (5) a palmaris profundus.

Paralysis of the anterior interosseous nerve in a supracondylar fracture is easily missed unless the distal phalanges of the thumb and the index finger are specifically examined for flexion power of the terminal joint. All other median nerve functions, sensory and motor, are intact. The injury is unrelated to the main median nerve trunk and does not implicate the median nerve at the fracture site. Volkmann's ischemia and anterior interosseous nerve paralysis are more likely to occur in fractures that are markedly displaced. Vascular obstruction usually occurs at the level of the fracture, and the presence of an anterior interosseous nerve paralysis has not been found to be a harbinger of Volkmann's ischemia.

In the six cases of anterior interosseous nerve paralysis that I have seen in children, spontaneous recovery occurred by the eighth week in all. Should clinical or electromyographic recovery not occur by this time, exploration of the median nerve from the distal part of the humerus through the pronator teres may be indicated.

A typical case is that of a 4-year-old boy who was admitted to the Lincoln Hospital in the Bronx on September 26, 1968, one hour after sustaining a supracondylar fracture of the left elbow with a posteroradial displacement of the distal fragment (Fig. 86B and C). There was moderate swelling and the radial pulse was palpable. The initial physician

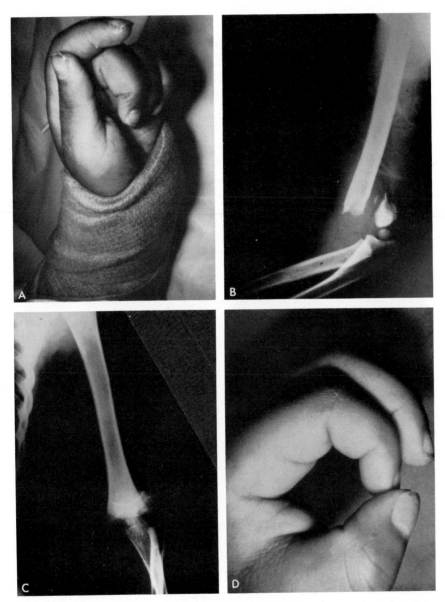

Figure 86.   *A*, Paralysis of the deep flexor of the thumb and the index finger. The patient could oppose the thumb and had normal sensation in the hand. *B* and *C*, Anteroposterior and lateral roentgenograms of the supracondylar fracture reveal the posterior and radial displacement. *D*, Full clinical postinjury recovery.

reported no muscular deficit in the hand although specific examination for the long flexor of the thumb and index finger was not recorded. Sensation was intact. An attempt at closed reduction of the fracture was unsuccessful and skeletal traction was applied with a Steinmann pin through the olecranon.

Four days later, under general anesthesia and with image intensifier monitoring during manipulation, closed reduction was again attempted. Satisfactory rotation alignment and reduction of the fracture could not be obtained and it was felt that soft tissue was interposed. An open reduction through a posterior approach was performed. Neither median nerve nor the brachial artery was visualized. Soft tissue was removed from the fracture gap. The fracture fragments were fixed with crossed Kirschner wires.

The postoperative examination of the patient revealed paralysis of the long flexor of the thumb and the index finger (Fig. 86A); that is, there was inability to flex the distal phalanx of these two digits. Clinically, the other muscles in the hand were normal, and sensation was intact. Examination at 2 weeks by electromyogram revealed fibrillations in the flexor pollicis longus and pronator quadratus. The pronator teres was normal. There were no fibrillations in the superficial flexors. Sensation was clinically intact and a ninhydrin test revealed normal sweating. For the next 5½ weeks there was no change, but then improvement commenced and by the eighth week full recovery had returned to both the index finger and the thumb.

The main median nerve trunk has been entrapped in fractures of the humerus, especially in the supracondylar region, and within the joint following elbow dislocation.[69, 72, 88, 89, 104] In this instance, there would be a complete high median nerve lesion. Early recognition and surgical management are of vital importance.

Volkmann's Ischemia. Patients with Volkmann's ischemia have muscle infarction which entraps the main median nerve and may involve the anterior interosseous branch separately. The flexor pollicis longus is at times part of the infarct. In one case without primary involvement of the flexor pollicis longus scar tissue compressed the anterior interosseous nerve proximally (Fig. 87E and F). There was also entrapment of the main median nerve trunk by a localized muscle infarct as it passed through the flexor superficialis arch. This case was seen late in the course of disease (about 2 years). The anterior interosseous nerve could be dissected out, as could the main median nerve trunk. Rather than risk failure of return of function of the flexor pollicis longus, the brachioradialis was used to motorize the flexor pollicis longus. The proximal end of the flexor profundus of the index finger was transferred into the flexor profundus of the fifth finger at the proper tension to obtain flexion of the index finger. Full flexion was obtained in all the digits (Fig. 87C and D). The anterior interosseous nerve was caught up in the same scarring process that involved the main median nerve and the ulnar nerve. The

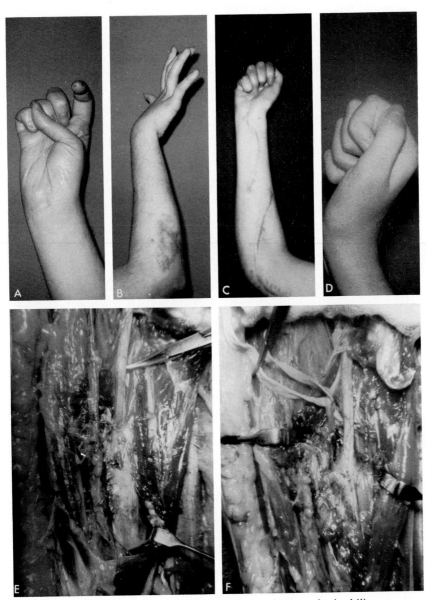

Figure 87.   *A* and *B*, Preoperative attitude of the hand. Note the inability to oppose the thumb or to flex the terminal phalanx of the thumb and index finger. In addition the fingers could be extended only when the wrist was flexed. *C* and *D*, Postoperatively the fingers could flex well. The brachioradialis was utilized to motorize the flexor pollicis longus. The adjacent functioning flexor profundus muscles motorized the deep flexor of the index finger. The fingers could flex and extend fully with the wrist in neutral position. *E*, The median nerve has been traced to the proximal end of the infarct. *F*, The anterior interosseous nerve under the rubber band is traced to the flexor pollicis longus.

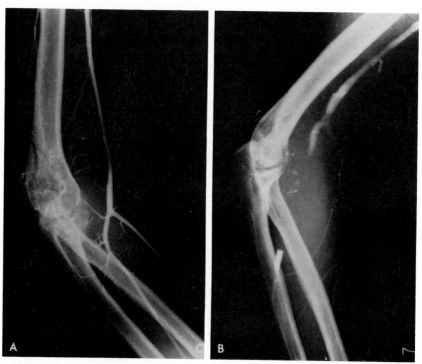

Figure 88. *A*, Arteriogram reveals the arterial tree to be intact but displaced anteriorly and compressed in the distal arm. *B*, Obstruction of the venous system in the region of the lacertus fibrosus is clearly seen.

flexor pollicis longus and the deep flexors of the index and long fingers were thus made nonfunctioning by local muscular infarction in addition to motor nerve entrapment. However, loss of function of the pronator quadratus was due to nerve entrapment rather than to muscle infarction.

In one case of impending Volkmann's ischemia it was noted that, as a result of a bullet penetrating the proximal forearm, the patient had paralysis of the flexor pollicis longus and the flexor profundus to the index and long fingers. In addition there was sensory loss in the median distribution of the hand. An arteriogram revealed an intact arterial tree but a venogram disclosed obstruction of the venous system in the region of the bullet wound under the lacertus (Fig. 88). A fasciotomy avoided major ischemia problems. The following day there was return of sensation to the median distribution of the hand and function to the anterior interosseous innervated structures. Therefore, there are occasions when both the anterior interosseous nerve and the main median nerve trunk can be involved in a compression phenomenon. When the compression involves the vascular tree, and venous return is obstructed, a secondary Volkmann's ischemia can be superimposed. It is interesting to note in this particular case that there was no pain on passive extension of the digits involved. This case may represent a borderline situation with initial nerve involvement rather than the usual primary muscle infarction of a Volkmann's ischemia typically with the nerve secondarily involved during the contracture phase of the ischemic process.

MANAGEMENT.   Based on all the cases of anterior interosseous nerve paralysis I have observed, along with my detailed anatomical dissections and review of the reported cases in the literature, the following conclusions are justified:

1. Patients with spontaneous paralysis of the anterior interosseous nerve should initially be treated by nonsurgical methods because many have a satisfactory return of function without recurrence. However, if there is no sign of clinical or electromyographic improvement in 6 to 8 weeks, or 12 weeks at the latest, exploration of the anterior interosseous nerve is indicated.

2. Patients who have a penetrating wound of the forearm and have an injury to the anterior interosseous nerve or to the anterior interosseous-fascicular component of the median nerve are best treated by primary exploration and repair if the condition of the wound and the general health of the patient are satisfactory.

3. If the anterior interosseous nerve is irreparable, appropriate muscle transfers should be performed. The flexor superficialis of the ring finger is an excellent motor for the flexor pollicis longus tendon. The brachioradialis is also a satisfactory substitute. The transfer of the proximal portion of the flexor profundus tendon of the index finger to the functioning profundus tendon of the ring or long finger at the wrist can provide satisfactory flexion of the distal phalanx of the index finger. In a recent case in which the flexor profundus muscles to both the index and long fingers were nonfunctioning, the extensor carpi radialis longus was rerouted over the radial border of the forearm and was found to be an excellent substitute.

Gantzer's Muscle

Gantzer's muscle,[33, 67] an accessory head to the flexor pollicis longus (Fig. 70), is found in approximately two-thirds of limbs and is innervated by the anterior interosseous nerve in the majority. Mangini,[67] in a detailed study of this muscle, demonstrated that it usually arose from the medial epicondyle of the humerus and inserted into the proximal part of the tendon of the flexor pollicis longus. It may have a double origin, the second arising from the coronoid process of the ulna. Kaplan[47] has noted that fibrosis with secondary contracture of this muscle can produce a flexion contracture of the thumb. In this instance there was a fibrous band extending from the medial epicondyle to the tendon of the flexor pollicis longus which normally inserts into the distal phalanx of the thumb.

In addition Gantzer's muscle may be a causative factor in an anterior interosseous nerve paralysis by fibrous entrapment.

Palmaris Profundus

The palmaris profundus, a muscle variation, takes origin from the deep fibro-osseous structures on the radial aspect of the proximal forearm.[91] The tendinous origin of the palmaris profundus arises in close proximity to the median nerve and its branches, located in this region. It inserts into the posterior aspect of the palmar aponeurosis, and its tendon passes through the carpal tunnel. When present, the tendinous origin could be a factor in producing an anterior interosseous nerve paralysis. Its distal tendon, which passes through the carpal tunnel, may be a contributing factor in median neuritis at the wrist (Fig. 89A).

Flexor Carpi Radialis Brevis

This variant muscle, like the palmaris profundus, arises from the deep fibro-osseous structures on the radial aspect of the proximal forearm (Fig. 89B). Its tendinous origin can also be a factor in the production of an anterior interosseous nerve syndrome. It inserts into the anterior aspect of the base of the second or third metacarpal. At the wrist its tendon passes through the same tunnel as the tendon of the flexor carpi radialis. In this region, I have seen it involved in both rheumatoid tenosynovitis and chronic traumatic tenosynovitis.

Pronator Syndrome

The pronator syndrome can be quite distinctive,[52, 53, 78, 96, 100] but so often it is elusive and difficult to diagnose with certainty. It is completely distinct from the anterior interosseous nerve syndrome.

It includes several elements, all of which, however, are rarely seen together so that the clinical picture of the pronator syndrome will vary and depend upon which of the following are present:

1. Pain in the proximal volar aspect of the forearm, increased by resistance to pronation of the forearm and flexion of the wrist (Fig. 90A).

2. Paresthesias in the radial 3½ digits.

3. A negative Phalen test (wrist flexion that does not produce median nerve paresthesia).

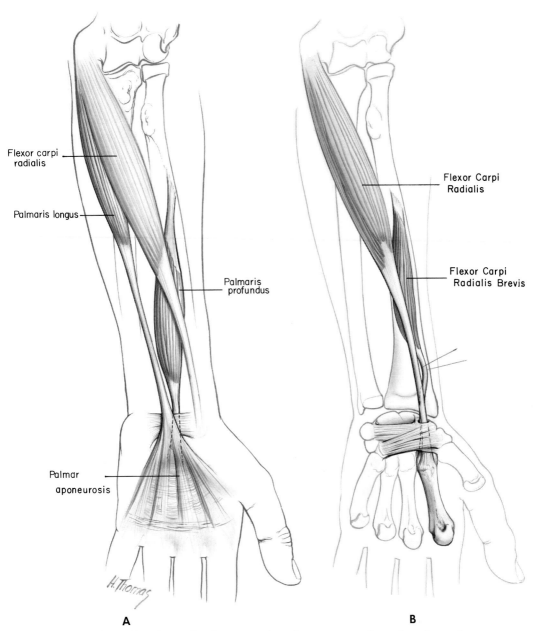

A

B

Figure 89. *A*, The palmaris profundus, a variant forearm muscle, arises from the junction of the middle and proximal radius and passes through the carpal tunnel. It inserts on the undersurface of the palmar aponeurosis. *B*, The flexor carpi radialis brevis, a variant forearm muscle, similarly, arises from the radius at the junction of its proximal and middle thirds. At the wrist level the anomalous tendon passes with the tendon of the flexor carpi radialis through a separate tunnel which is lateral to the carpal tunnel. The anomalous tendon inserts into the base of the second or third metacarpal bone.

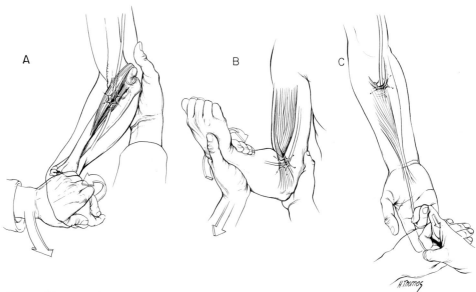

Figure 90.   *A*, Pain in the proximal forearm increased by resistance to pronation of the forearm and flexion of the wrist is a positive sign of median nerve compression at the level of the pronator teres. *B*, Pain in the proximal forearm increased by resistance to forearm supination and elbow flexion is a positive sign for compression of the median nerve at the lacertus fibrosus. *C*, Pain in the proximal forearm reproduced by resistance to flexion of the flexor superficialis of the long finger is a positive sign for compression of the median nerve at the flexor digitorum superficialis arch.

   4. Variable weakness of the median-innervated intrinsic muscles.

   5. Normal function of the extrinsic muscles innervated by the anterior interosseous nerve (flexor pollicis longus, flexor profundus muscles to the index and long fingers and the pronator quadratus).

   6. Localized EMG abnormalities with sensory or motor conduction delay in the proximal forearm. Abnormal electromyographic activity findings of muscles sampled consisting of fibrillations, positive sharp waves, loss of motor units and increase of polyphasics have been described.[11] The specific median nerve–innervated muscles found to have these abnormalities are supplied distal to the pronator teres.

   Although it is true that the syndrome is caused to the greatest extent by compression of the median nerve at the pronator level, there are two other areas of potential entrapment in close vicinity in the proximal forearm. These are at the lacertus fibrosus and the flexor superficialis bridge. Reproduction of the forearm pain when elbow flexion and forearm supination are resisted suggests that the compression is at the lacertus level (Fig. 90*B*). Forearm pain reproduced by resistance to flexion of the long finger flexor superficialis localizes the pathology to the superficialis bridge (Fig. 90*C*).

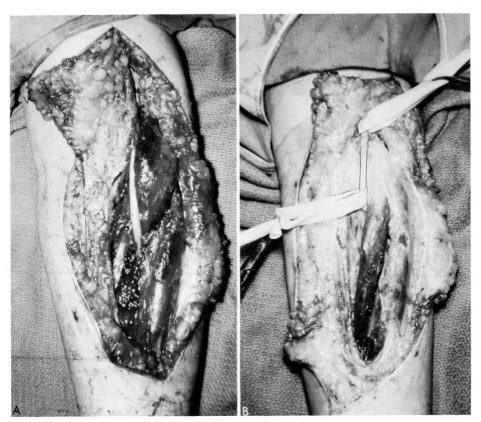

Figure 91. *A*, Left forearm of a 15-year-old girl with a pronator syndrome. The pronator teres was markedly hypertrophied. It was translocated posterior to the median nerve. *B*, A 44-year-old female with a pronator syndrome of the left forearm. The pronator was of normal size. A neurolysis of the median nerve (two Penrose) was performed. Note the usual size of the pronator teres.

The anatomical abnormalities that have been observed with this entity are:

1. Hypertrophied pronator teres (Fig. 91).
2. Fibrous bands within the pronator teres.
3. Median nerve passing posterior to both heads of the pronator teres.
4. Thickened lacertus fibrosus.
5. Thickened flexor superficialis arch (Fig. 92).
6. An accessory tendinous origin of the flexor carpi radialis from the ulna.

The following case presents an example of the difficulty in diagnosing this syndrome. A 45-year-old white cab driver sustained a comminuted fracture of the radial head. It was excised within the first 48 hours (Fig. 93*A*). His elbow was immobilized for 3 weeks in a plaster cast in a func-

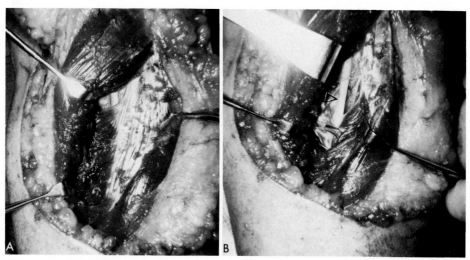

Figure 92.   *A*, The flexor superficialis arch is seen crossing the median nerve. The flexor carpi radialis is retracted. *B*, The flexor superficialis arch has been excised. Note the narrowed median nerve (open arrow). There are vessels crossing under the flexor superficialis arch. If thrombosed they could be an additional factor in the pathogenesis of the pronator syndrome.

tional position after the operative procedure. Subsequently, he developed vague pain in the elbow and forearm. Within a few months subjective paresthesias in the radial three fingers of the hand gradually became apparent. Objectively, sensation was identical in the index and little fingers. The involved hand showed more redness than the opposite hand. As the elbow motion increased, the pain and numbness of his limb increased. A persistent lack of 30 degrees of full extension of the elbow was noted.

At first the localization of the median nerve dysfunction was not clear because EMG studies on two occasions were completely normal — no conduction delay and no fibrillations of the thenar muscles were evident. Wrist roentgenograms revealed mild settling of the distal radioulnar joint (suggesting, perhaps, the initial injury was of the Essex-Lopresti type fracture-dislocation), thereby further complicating the localization of the median nerve entrapment (Fig. 93*B*). The Phalen wrist flexion test was negative. The Tinel sign became positive in the volar aspect of the proximal forearm. The patient did not improve with conservative measures.

Exploration of the median nerve through the region of the pronator teres revealed the median nerve passing deep to both heads of this muscle rather than through it (Fig. 93*C* and *D*). The nerve lacked its usual markings in this region. The pronator was lengthened, the arch of the flexor superficialis was divided, and the median nerve was rerouted

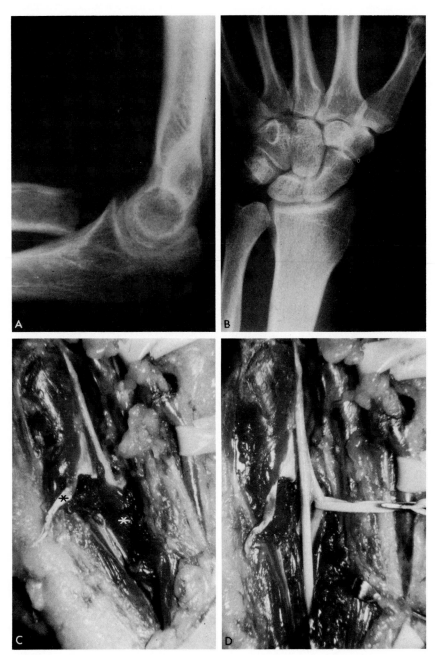

Figure 93. *A*, The left radial head has been completely excised. *B*, Anteroposterior roentgenogram of the left wrist reveals mild settling of the distal radioulnar joint. *C*, The tendon of the pronator teres (black *) has been lengthened. The median nerve is seen passing deep to the deep head of the pronator teres (white *). *D*, The rubber band is retracting the anterior interosseous nerve. The median nerve has been freed. There is a difference in the color of the median nerve deep to the pronator teres when compared to the more proximal portion of the median nerve trunk and its anterior interosseous nerve branch.

subcutaneously. This was accomplished by resuturing the lengthened pronator teres posterior to the median nerve.

Postoperatively, the patient had an excellent recovery. His complaints subsided and he regained the extension movement at the elbow. He returned to his usual work as a cab driver 6 weeks after the nerve exploration, and 6 months after sustaining the fracture.

A pronator syndrome can be insidious in its development and may be present in spite of normal electrical studies. EMG studies when positive are an aid in confirming the diagnosis, but negative findings should not deter a necessary nerve exploration. Only subjective sensory findings in the median nerve distribution of the hand may be present. A sympathetic outflow disturbance may be a component of the symptomatology.

I have observed that in the middle and, especially, the last trimester of pregnancy this syndrome may be found. One young lady had a carpal tunnel syndrome on one side and a pronator syndrome on the opposite. Interestingly, only the conduction studies on the carpal tunnel side were abnormal. The pronator syndrome responded to a local injection[96] of xylocaine and steroid, while the opposite wrist required release of the carpal tunnel.

Several cases of entrapment of the median nerve due to the restraining effect of the lacertus fibrosus have had an acute course. This pattern of entrapment usually occurs in patients on renal dialysis or anticoagulant therapy, the common history being that a blood sample was drawn from the antecubital fossa with difficulty. Intense and neuritic pain promptly develop in the forearm. Numbness and dysesthesias of the radial 3½ fingers follow rapidly. If the situation is left untreated, a high median nerve paralysis rapidly ensues (Fig. 94A). Prompt surgical exploration (preferably before the paralysis develops) with release of the lacertus fibrosus and any other obstructing fibrous structure, along with evacuation of the hematoma, is indicated (Fig. 94B–D). Delayed management leads to prolonged discomfort, parethesias, paresis or paralysis. Prompt surgical intervention is necessary to obtain maximal improvement.

Bell and Goldner,[5] reporting on children with cerebral palsy who have pronation contractures of the forearm, state that forced immobilization in a long-arm plaster cast in supination can lead to median nerve dysfunction. The tight fascia and shortened muscles are believed to be the causative factor in production of the symptoms. Prompt removal of the cast usually relieves the symptoms.

Carpal Tunnel Syndrome

This relatively common entrapment syndrome[87] is most often caused by narrowing of the carpal tunnel, but it can be caused by enlargement of

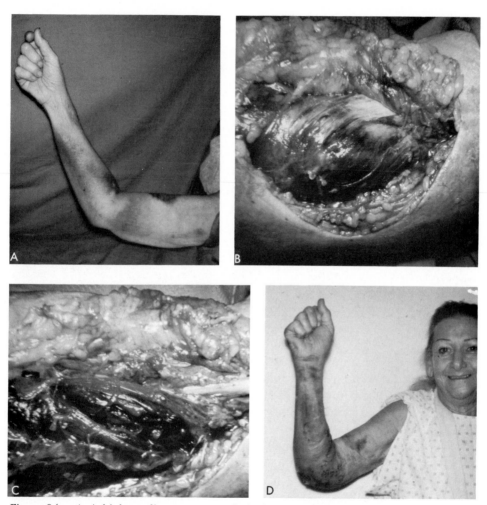

Figure 94.   *A*, A high median nerve paralysis due to acute lacertus fibrosus syndrome secondary to venipuncture from the antecubital fossa in a 59-year-old female who was anticoagulated for renal dialysis. *B*, Surgery was performed within a few hours of the development of symptoms of pain and numbness. The lacertus fibrosus is seen with the tense hematoma in the pronator teres muscle. *C*, The lacertus fibrosus has been incised and the median nerve liberated. The hematoma under the lacertus and within the pronator teres has been evacuated. *D*, Within two days the paralysis and numbness subsided. The patient was pain-free immediately after surgery.

the median nerve. The condition is most frequently seen in female patients between 40 and 60 years of age, although it can be seen in children and older patients. Pain, numbness and paresthesias occur in the distal median nerve distribution of the hand — usually the radial 3½ digits. Nocturnal burning pain in the hand, which is relieved by shaking the hand, is frequently reported.

The diagnosis of carpal tunnel syndrome is readily made when the entire spectrum of signs and symptoms is present: numbness in the appropriate digits, atrophy of the thenar muscles, a positive Phalen sign, increased symptomatology with inflation of an arm tourniquet above venous pressure, and motor and sensory electroneuromyographic distal median nerve abnormalities. The complete clinical spectrum may not be present, and it is not unusual to observe atypical findings. Numbness restricted to the long finger, absence of muscle atrophy, a negative Phalen or Tinel sign, normal electromyographic studies, pain in the shoulder, sensitivity to cold, or reflex dystrophy frequently becloud the diagnostic picture.

When the presenting symptom is pain in the shoulder, an unusual site for a carpal tunnel syndrome to manifest itself, knowledge of this should suggest to the treating physician that he examine the wrist and the shoulder.[11, 18, 55] A diagnosis of carpal tunnel syndrome should not be excluded because of symptoms in the proximal upper extremity. The clinical suspicion that the pathology is at the wrist, involving the median nerve, can be confirmed with the EMG. In past years, when standard EMG methods were used, 25 per cent of patients with this syndrome had normal studies. However, newer techniques, which compare digit to palm and palm to wrist, offer greater accuracy and confirmation.[11] It has been suggested that pain in the arm proximal to the wrist is related to inability of the median nerve to move freely in a longitudinal direction because of proximal median nerve fixation at the neck, thoracic outlet or arm.[75]

Personal observations reveal that half of the patients with carpal tunnel syndrome respond to conservative treatment measures. Splinting of the wrist in a neutral position combined with use of a diuretic is effective in these patients. Any underlying systemic disease should be brought under control if possible. Local injections of steroid and xylocaine into the carpal tunnel, although recommended by some, are not favored by this author. If relief is not obtained by conservative methods, surgical release of the transverse carpal ligament should be undertaken.[19] Specific indications such as thenar atrophy, prolonged symptomatology with markedly delayed conduction values, and the appearance of the nerve at surgery require internal neurolysis.[20] When I perform an internal neurolysis it is limited to clinically involved funiculi, as, for example, the thenar branch when there is atrophy, and the few medial funiculi within the nerve that are destined for the second and third web spaces when the long finger is markedly symptomatic.

A satisfactory exposure is obtained by an incision on the ulnar side of the carpal tunnel, step-cutting at the wrist and extending the incision on the ulnar side of the distal forearm. A transverse wrist incision is not utilized. During the procedure, care must be taken to preserve the median palmar cutaneous nerve. Injury to this nerve can result in post-operative pain.[15, 110]

Direct trauma, pregnancy, menopausal hormone changes and local tumors (ganglia, lipoma) have been most frequently linked with this entity. Systemic diseases, such as hypothyroidism, pleonosteosis, amyloidosis, gout, myeloma, rheumatoid disease and diabetes, have also been significantly associated causative factors.

From time to time anatomical variant structures have been reported as a factor in the symptomatology. These anatomical variants pass through the fibro-osseous tunnel on the volar aspect of the wrist through which the median nerve passes to reach the palm. The palmaris profundus, variant flexor superficialis muscles, variant lumbrical muscles, and enlarged median artery are to be noted.

Reimann et al.[91] noted the *palmaris profundus* as one of the many variations of the palmaris longus. The palmaris profundus arises from the radius, ulna and interosseous membrane in the proximal forearm and inserts into the dorsal aspect of the palmar aponeurosis. It passes through the carpal tunnel. It can produce symptoms if its tendon is large or its musculotendinous junction extends beneath the carpal tunnel. Ashby[1] has reported the association of a hypertrophied palmaris longus muscle in the distal forearm with median neuritic complaints which required excision of the anomalous muscle.

Variations of the flexor superficialis muscles are not uncommon.[14,31,37,66] There are frequently accessory tendons and cross communications between the tendons of the ring and little fingers.[49] Of greater significance, the muscle of the flexor superficialis may extend well into the palm,[115,117] thus crowding the median nerve at the wrist. This arrangement is the usual finding in the lizard. I have seen one flexor superficialis which was digastric; the short connecting tendon was located at the level of the carpal tunnel. Case[14] reported one such occurrence, which presented as a pseudotumor of the palm. Other pseudotumors of the palm have been reported by Wesser et al.[117] and Vichare[115] in which the entire flexor superficialis of the index finger was fleshy well into the palm. Butler and Bigley[13] reported an anomalous index lubrical tendinous origin from the flexor superficialis in association with this syndrome.

There is considerable difference in recommended treatment of these pseudotumors, from leaving them in place, to excising them, to shaving the muscle down. However, once the carpal tunnel is released, the symptoms usually subside, regardless of the surgical management of the variant muscular structure.

The *median artery*, which lies anterior to the median nerve, can become enlarged and at times can cause neuritic symptoms. It may on rare occasion be involved in a pathological process, such as giant cell arteritis[12] or aneurysm formation, and cause the symptoms of median nerve irritation. On occasion the enlarged median artery may form the major arterial tree of the hand.[22] Rarely, it may be the only supply to the index and long fingers. It therefore behooves the treating physician in the appropriate case to evaluate the arterial supply of the hand before sacrificing the enlarged median artery. Release of the carpal tunnel in and of itself can relieve the symptoms.

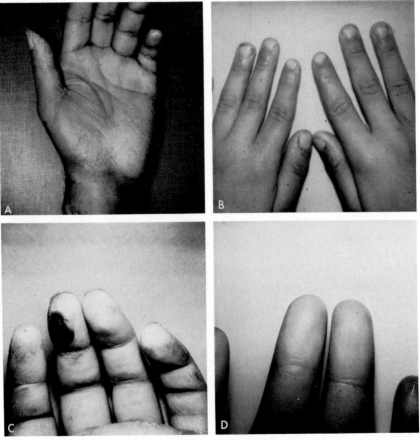

Figure 95.   *A*, Left hand. Partial median nerve and complete ulnar nerve sensory loss. The basilar area of the thenar eminence (median palmar cutaneous nerve) and the thumb are anesthetic. In addition the entire ulnar sensory region, the hypothenar eminence, the little finger and the ulnar half of the ring finger are anesthetic. *B*, Note the diminished size of the left index finger of a child with a carpal tunnel syndrome. *C*, Trophic ulcer in the long finger in a median nerve palsy due to a fracture of the wrist which resolved following median nerve neurolysis (*D*).

Carpal tunnel syndrome has also been caused by other less common etiological factors, such as insertion of an artificial tendon, retraction of a lacerated flexor profundus tendon from a digit, and mycobacterial infection of the synovium of the flexor tendons.

Gardner[34] described a pseudocarpal tunnel syndrome with the entrapment of the median nerve at the lower end of the flexor superficialis, 4 to 5 cm. proximal to the transverse carpal ligament. His case followed an injury with local tenderness and firmness of the soft tissues just proximal to the wrist.

Children with carpal tunnel syndrome can present with atrophy of the soft tissues of the index finger (Fig. 95B). Lettin[60] first noted diminution in size of the index finger in a juvenile with a carpal tunnel syndrome.

Injuries about the wrist with injury to the median nerve may result in a trophic ulcer of a digit which can resolve following release of the carpal tunnel and neurolysis (Fig. 95C and D).

The Thenar Motor Branch of the Median Nerve

The median nerve usually enters the carpal tunnel as one unit. This corresponds to the volar flexion crease of the wrist. Within the epineural sheath of the median nerve the terminal funiculi are well organized at this level. They are arranged linearly according to their destination. The motor fibers are anterior, and the funiculi for each of the web spaces and the lateral 3½ digits are lined up from lateral to medial in progressive sequence within the nerve.[108, 109] At the distal end of the flexor retinaculum the median nerve usually divides into two terminal branches. From the radial division the thenar branch classically arises and takes a recurrent course just distal to the flexor retinaculum (Fig. 96A). The thenar branch usually traverses this extraligamentous course. The lateral and medial side of the thumb and the lateral side of the index finger receive their sensory distribution from this radial division of the median nerve. The ulnar component of the median nerve supplies the second and third web spaces and their corresponding digits. The digital nerves supply the lumbricales as they pass them. The radial two lumbricales, occasionally the third, and rarely the fourth, are innervated by these branches.

The thenar branch can arise under the flexor retinaculum, a subligamentous origin, from the median nerve from its lateral side and can pass in a recurrent course about the distal edge of the retinaculum (Fig. 96B and C). The median nerve can bifurcate into its two major divisions within the carpal tunnel. In this instance, the recurrent thenar branch usually arises from the lateral division deep to the flexor retinaculum (Fig. 96C).

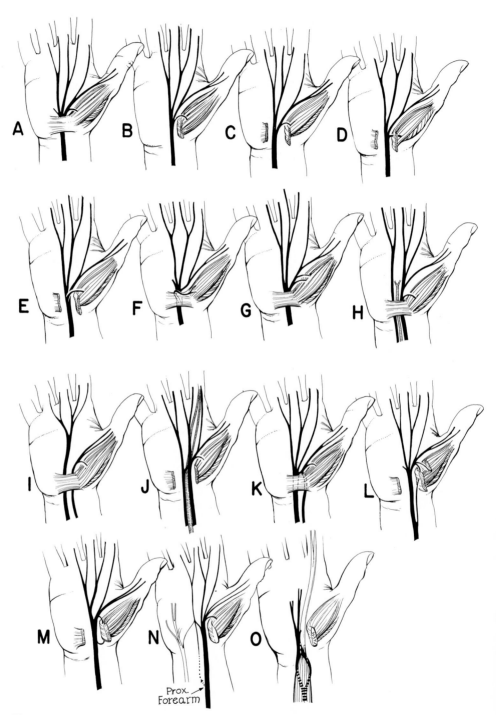

Figure 96.   Variations of the median nerve and its thenar branch at the level of the carpal tunnel (see text for details and clinical significance).

Frequently, the thenar branch passes through a separate tunnel in the flexor retinaculum 2 to 6 mm. from its distal margin (Fig. 96D).[46, 84]

When the motor branch arises under this ligament it usually does so on the radial or anteroradial aspect of the nerve; however, this motor branch may arise from the ulnar side of the median nerve within the carpal tunnel (Fig. 96E and F).[24, 38, 57, 58, 70] Associated hypertrophy of the superficial head of the flexor pollicis brevis or the palmaris brevis, or both, has been described in these cases. The thenar branch, which arises from the ulnar aspect of the median nerve, can pass aberrantly through this muscle mass anterior to the flexor retinaculum (Fig. 96F).[70]

There can be more than one motor thenar branch (Fig. 96G). Two and three branches have been observed.[38, 57, 58, 61] These traveled either in their usual recurrent course or via an aberrant path. On occasion an accessory motor branch can arise in the distal forearm or proximal wrist. It can pass through the carpal tunnel or through the flexor retinaculum (Fig. 96K–M).[57, 58, 61, 82] Thus, motor neural fibers to the thenar muscles can travel through their usual course and through an ancillary proximal branch. Electrical stimulation of these variant branches, using a bipolar electrode, is important when evaluating their true function — sensory, motor or mixed (Fig. 97).

A persistent median artery (Fig. 96H) can be associated with high division of the median nerve.[23, 41, 57, 58] Variant muscles such as an aberrant flexor digitorum superficialis (Fig. 96O)[3] or a lumbrical (Fig. 96J)[95] can also be associated with high division of this peripheral nerve. Therefore, limited exposure at the wrist level may not reveal vessel or muscle variants in association with high division of the median nerve (Fig. 96I).[50]

Finally, the thenar branch can be absent. This is observed in the "all-ulnar hand," in which the entire thenar muscle group is supplied by the ulnar nerve via anastomotic pathways through the entire limb.[9, 93]

Variations of the motor branch of the thenar muscles are numerous. Knowledge of these is of importance to the treating physician, electromyographer, and neurologist.

If the palmaris brevis or the superficial head of the flexor pollicis brevis is enlarged when observed during carpal tunnel surgery, then special care must be taken to avoid injury to an aberrant origin of the motor branch from the ulnar side of the nerve rather than the radial. This hypertrophied muscle is located anterior to the flexor retinaculum. When this muscle variant is found, it is necessary to identify the median nerve within the carpal tunnel. Its motor branch should be identified by opening the carpal tunnel on its medial side. The motor branch is then traced distally as it recurs through the superficial hypertrophied muscle (Fig. 96F).[70]

As has been noted, the motor branch may pierce the flexor retinaculum 2 to 6 mm. proximal to the distal border of this structure. In this way, a distinct tunnel for the recurrent nerve in the distal retinaculum can exist. It has clinical significance because a carpal tunnel syndrome may present at times with more motor or even pure motor dysfunction than the usual sensory median nerve disturbance. It is important to release this entrapped nerve branch before the motor weakness of the thumb has been present for more than 12 to 18 months. The length of time for possible recovery depends upon the degree of atrophy and the extent of neural damage. Sensory paresthesias usally are improved or relieved by release of the carpal tunnel. The recurrent branch, however, may have to be traced through the flexor retinaculum into the thenar musculature when this anatomical variation is present.

When dealing with lacerations of the motor branch of the median nerve, knowledge of variations in the number of branches and their variant courses is of vital importance, for it may be necessary to repair not one but two of these branches (Fig. 96G and M). Similarly, when there is aberrant high passage of the motor branch proximal to the wrist, a laceration of this branch, but not involving the main median nerve trunk, can cause loss of opposition of the thumb (Fig. 96K–M). When there is dual innervation of the thenar muscles, laceration of the thenar recurrent branch may present clinically with only weakness of opposition of the thumb.

Finally, in an "all ulnar nerve-innervated hand" there is absence of a thenar branch from the median nerve. Sensation to the hand is also significantly altered because the median nerve may supply only the volar aspect of the index finger. In this case, with a complete median nerve laceration at the wrist, only a small median nerve is found in the carpal tunnel. All of the usual sensory and motor funiculi carried within the median nerve have had an aberrant passage to their sensory and motor end organs. Knowledge of these variations is of prime importance to the operating surgeon.

High Division of the Median Nerve

High division of the median nerve can occur at the level of the wrist or forearm (Fig. 96H, I, J, and N). The two components of the median nerve in the carpal tunnel can be of equal or unequal size — either the medial (Fig. 96I) or the lateral component (Fig. 96N) may be larger. It would not be proper to call this anatomical finding a "reduplication" of the nerve because the median nerve has not been duplicated; rather, high division has occurred. This high division can occur with a small or large ellipse.[42] Within the center of the ellipse is muscle, tendon or blood vessels.

One such high division presented itself during a cadaver dissection.[119] In addition to the high division the limb had multiple neural

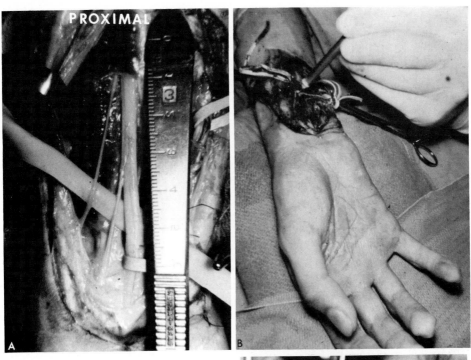

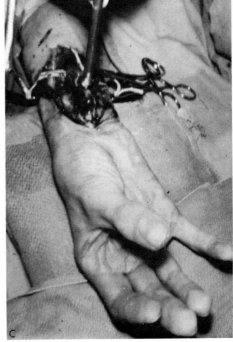

Figure 97. *A*, The median nerve with two branches arising from the medial side of the distal right forearm. *B*, A bipolar electrode is applied to the more distal branch without applying the current. The thumb is noted on the skeletal plane of the hand. *C*, The thumb is noted to abduct with application of the current. This indicates that some of the motor fibers to the thenar muscles pass through this variant pathway. A similar response was obtained by stimulating the median nerve distal to the takeoff of these branches. This suggests that motor fibers to the thenar muscles in this instance travel via two pathways, one through the median nerve, and the other through an accessory high-rising branch.

variants: a Martin-Gruber anastomosis, a communication between the ulnar and median nerve distal to the flexor retinaculum, and two components to the median nerve traversing the lower half of the forearm and carpal tunnel.

A dissection of the right upper limb revealed a high origin of a branch to the third web space of the hand (Fig. 98). The branch arose 9½ cm. distal to the medial epicondyle, which was 4 cm. distal to the origin of the anterior interosseous branch of the median nerve. It penetrated the flexor digitorum superficialis 2½ cm. distal to the flexor superficialis arch. It arose from the anterior aspect of the median nerve and ran through the muscular mass of the flexor digitorum superficialis obliquely for 2 cm. (Fig. 98A and C). This variant branch then came to lie partially under the cover of the flexor carpi radialis at its musculocutaneous junction (Fig. 98C and D). In the midforearm the anomalous branch lay in a groove on the anterior surface of the flexor superficialis between the long and index finger portions. More distally, it was covered only by a thin layer of the antibrachial fascia. At the level of the carpal tunnel the nerve passed beneath the transverse carpal ligament medial to the main trunk of the median nerve. One and one-half cm. distal to the transverse carpal ligament, a small branch from the main median nerve crossed obliquely ulnarward to join the aberrant branch to the third web space. A similar communication was found to arise from the ulnar nerve branch to the fourth web space at the end of the transverse carpal ligament, where it also joined the aberrant branch to the third web space (Fig. 98B–D). In addition, a Martin-Gruber anastomosis from the anterior interosseous branch of the median nerve to the ulnar nerve was found in the proximal forearm. This neural anastomosis between the median and ulnar nerves in the proximal forearm followed a course parallel and just distal to the ulnar artery and vein.

Sunderland notes that Gruber in 1870 reported four specimens in which the branch to the third web space arose in the proximal forearm instead of in the palm.[109] Hartmann reported a similar anatomical specimen.[42]

The clinical significance of such variations is clear: Such aberrant nerves could be inadvertently injured or traumatized during carpal tunnel surgery. These variant branches are particularly vulnerable during flexor tenosynovectomy. Furthermore, the unusual course of the variant branch anterior to the flexor digitorum superficialis in the distal half of the forearm exposes it to potential damage during surgery in this region. Adequate incisions and wider exposure at the wrist and forearm would help to identify these variant neural structures in order to avoid unnecessary complications.

The carpal tunnel syndrome, with its classically observed sensory pattern of pain and numbness of the radial 3½ digits, can vary on occasion.

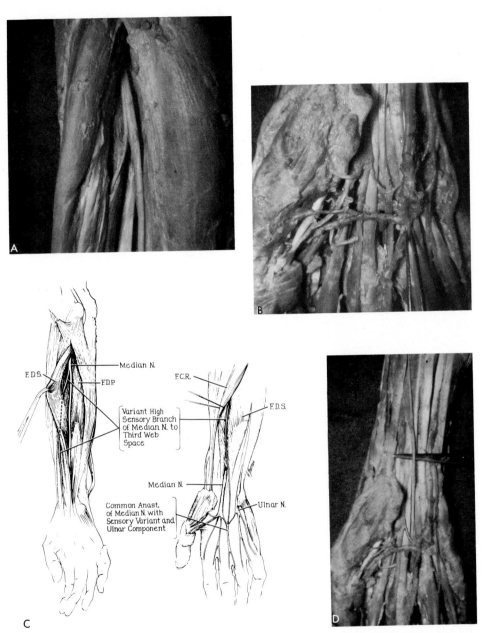

Figure 98. *A*, At the junction of the proximal and middle thirds of the forearm, the variant sensory branch is seen penetrating the flexor superficialis muscle 2 cm. distal to its takeoff from the median nerve. *B*, Closeup of the wrist, demonstrating the main median nerve trunk and the variant sensory branch passing through the carpal tunnel. *C*, A composite artist drawing of an anomalous high sensory branch of the median nerve to the third web space in a right forearm. *D*, The variant sensory branch of the median nerve is on the hemostat. It is seen passing superficial to the flexor superficialis from under cover of the flexor carpi radialis in the midforearm.

Isolated symptoms referable to only the third web space or the ulnar side of the long finger as the earliest sign of a carpal tunnel entrapment may be noted; conversely, the symptoms may involve only the more lateral component of the median nerve, sparing the third web space. This finding should cause the examiner to consider the possibility of this variation. Similarly, lacerations of the forearm associated with numbness of the third web space and its accompanying digital manifestations in the ulnar half of the long finger and radial half of the ring finger suggest the occurrence of this anomaly.

Martin-Gruber Anastomosis

The Martin-Gruber anastomosis,[39, 71] for the most part, carries motor fibers from the median nerve or its branches to the ulnar nerve in the forearm in two ways:

1. From the median nerve trunk in the proximal forearm to the ulnar nerve in the middle to distal third of the forearm.

2. From the anterior interosseous nerve branch of the median nerve to the ulnar nerve in the middle to distal third of the forearm (Fig. 74).

There is yet another anastomosis between the median and ulnar nerve branches within the flexor digitorum profundus muscle in the midforearm. This determines the degree of partial or complete innervation of the deep flexors of the digits by either the median or the ulnar nerve.

An extremely rare type of cross innervation in the forearm which brings ulnar funiculi to the median nerve is exemplified by one of Rowntree's recorded cases.[93] A complete lesion of the ulnar nerve at the wrist did not present with an ulnar clawed hand. Stimulation of the ulnar nerve at the elbow produced good contractions of the interosseous, adductor pollicis, and hypothenar muscles. I have seen one identical case with a complete ulnar nerve laceration at the wrist manifesting an ulnar claw hand only after the ulnar nerve was blocked at the elbow level.

The clinical significance of the Martin-Gruber anastomosis has been referred to previously in the discussion of variations of the anterior interosseous nerve syndrome. It is also of importance in the understanding of the function of the hand following high ulnar nerve injury.

This anastomosis carries the motor supply to many of the intrinsic muscles of the hand (first, second, third dorsal interosseous, hypothenar, and, at times, the adductor pollicis muscles). With a complete lesion of the ulnar nerve proximal to the anastomosis many of the intrinsic muscles will function through this anatomical variation. In an extreme case, with a complete high ulnar nerve lesion, it is possible to have no gross visible ulnar motor loss in the hand. Sensory loss in the ring and little fingers may be the only deficit.

Likewise, in a complete high median nerve laceration at or above the elbow, there may be a high median nerve loss in the hand, but in addition some of the intrinsic muscles may be partially or completely paralyzed. The ulnar nerve need not be injured in this instance. A possible clue to this occurrence is the presence of normal sensation in the ring and little fingers. Thus a complete median nerve lesion at the elbow can present with a typical high median nerve hand paralysis in addition to intrinsic muscle loss.

An extreme example is the "all median nerve hand" in which the median nerve through this anastomosis could present with a hand having only extension of the digits and wrist. In this type of hand there may be sensation only in the fifth finger.

Accessory Motor Supply to the Flexor Superficialis

The flexor superficialis motor supply has several variations. Accessory nerves to the flexor superficialis arise at times from the flexor carpi radialis or palmaris longus motor branch and follow a course between the superficial and deep head of the pronator teres. This accessory branch then goes deep to the flexor superficialis arch to innervate a portion of the superficialis muscle mass. Similarly, the anterior interosseous nerve, which supplies the flexor pollicis longus, the medial half of the flexor profundus and the pronator quadratus, can at times supply a portion of the flexor superficialis. Likewise, when a Martin-Gruber anastomosis occurs between the median and ulnar nerves in the forearm, it arises frequently from the anterior interosseous nerve (Fig. 74). This has been reported to occur in 8 of 100 upper limb specimens. An accessory motor branch to the distal half of the flexor superficialis to the index finger is found at the junction of the middle and distal thirds of the forearm in 45 per cent of limbs.[8]

These particular variations are of clinical importance because they help to explain how the flexor superficialis muscle is spared to some extent when the main median nerve trunk is completely severed just proximal to its major branches to the flexor superficialis in the region of the flexor arch.

Median Palmar Cutaneous Nerve

The median palmar cutaneous nerve usually arises from the radial side of the median nerve 5.5 cm. proximal to the radial styloid. It passes distally to the ulnar aspect of the flexor carpi radialis tendon sheath (Figs. 99A, 100, 101B–D). At the level of the proximal end of the carpal tunnel

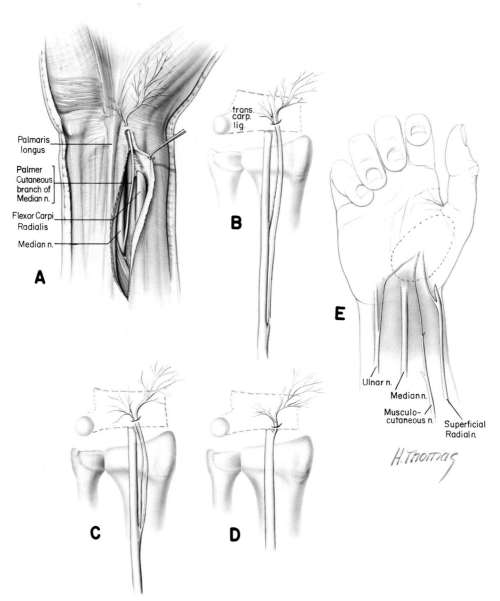

Figure 99.   *A,* The usual course of the palmar cutaneous branch of the median nerve is depicted in this right wrist. Note the tunnel in the transverse carpal ligament, through which it passes, and its two terminal major branches. *B,* The median palmar cutaneous nerve can be double. An additional branch can arise more proximally or both can take origin at the usual level (*C*). *D,* It can also have a low takeoff from the median nerve. It then directly penetrates the flexor retinaculum. *E,* The median palmar cutaneous branch of the median nerve can be absent. The skin of the thenar eminence is then supplied by either a branch of the superficial radial nerve, an anterior division of the musculocutaneous nerve, the palmar cutaneous branch of the ulnar nerve or a combination of these branches.

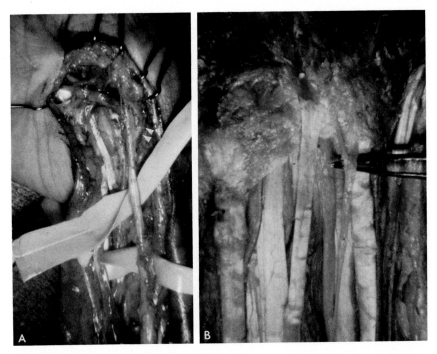

Figure 100.   *A,* The median nerve (Penrose drains) is noted to the extreme radial side of the carpal tunnel of this right wrist. It is tethered by the median palmar cutaneous nerve (two white arrows) in a case of juvenile Volkmann's ischemia due to a Factor VII deficiency. The wrist had been deformed and fixed in marked flexion and ulnar deviation. *B,* Right cadaver specimen demonstrating the details of the median palmar cutaneous nerve (hemostat).

this nerve passes through a short tunnel of its own, 9 to 16 mm. within the transverse carpal ligament.[110] At this level the median palmar cutaneous nerve divides into two major branches, medial and lateral, which subsequently ramify to innervate the skin of the thenar eminence (Fig. 95*A*). The lateral branch is usually larger (Fig. 99*A*).

VARIATIONS OF THE MEDIAN PALMAR CUTANEOUS NERVE.   The median palmar cutaneous nerve has significant variations. There can be two separate median palmar cutaneous nerves, one arising at the usual location, the other arising from the median nerve at 9 cm. or even higher in the proximal forearm (Fig. 99*B*).[109]

The two terminals may divide more proximally than the region of distal flexion crease of the wrist. When this occurs, two major branches — two median palmar cutaneous nerves — can arise from the median nerve 5.5 cm. proximal to the radial styloid.[43] These two branches can arise from a common trunk at this level (Fig. 99*C*).

The median palmar cutaneous nerve has been observed to arise from the median nerve at the more distal level of the radial styloid, or just beyond, within the proximal end of carpal tunnel. It penetrates the

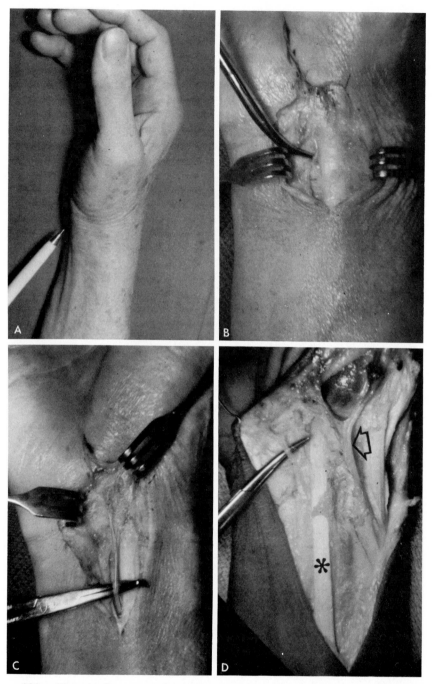

Figure 101.   Chronic flexor carpi radialis tendinitis of the right wrist. *A*, Note the swelling at the distal end of the right wrist in the terminal portion of the flexor carpi radialis. *B*, The median palmar cutaneous nerve is noted in the thickened flexor carpi radialis sheath on its ulnar side. *C*, The sheath has been released. The nerve has been traced to its terminal branches. *D*, Another right wrist demonstrating both the median palmar cutaneous nerve (hemostat) and the superficial radial nerve (arrow) prior to reconstruction of the thumb metacarpocarpal joint with a portion of the flexor carpi radialis tendon (Littler-Eaton procedure). The median palmar cutaneous nerve is on the ulnar side of the flexor carpi radialis (*).

flexor retinaculum and palmar aponeurosis to supply the thenar skin area (Fig. 99D).

The palmar branch of the median nerve may be absent,[109] being replaced by either the anterior division of the musculocutaneous nerve, a branch of the superficial radial nerve, a branch of the palmar cutaneous nerve from the ulnar nerve or a combination of these branches (Fig. 99E).[59]

Finally, adjacent to the wrist flexion crease, the palmaris longus tendon may have a broad insertion or a variant muscular attachment. Thus, the palmaris longus tendon or muscle can be observed in juxtaposition with or covering this sensory branch.

CLINICAL SIGNIFICANCE OF THE VARIATIONS OF THE MEDIAN PALMAR CUTANEOUS NERVE. A neuroma of this sensory branch can be distressing.[15] If two median palmar cutaneous branches are present, there may be two neuromas. Removal of one would leave the patient with persistent symptoms. When a patient demonstrates two points of pain on direct percussion, the likelihood is that two neuromas are present.

Entrapment of the median palmar cutaneous nerve has been described. When the condition is clinically apparent, release of the compressing structure is indicated. An anomalous palmaris longus muscle associated with pain and numbness in the thenar eminence has been reported.[105]

When the median palmar cutaneous nerve is absent, then the anterior division of the musculocutaneous nerve, the superficial radial nerve and the palmar cutaneous branch of the ulnar nerve assume greater clinical significance. These nerves are vulnerable to laceration because of their subcutaneous course in the distal forearm and hand. When variations of the median palmar cutaneous nerve are present, an enlarged area of sensory denervation can be noted when one of these sensory branches is injured. For example, if the superficial radial nerve supplies the skin of the thenar eminence as well as its usual dorsal aspect of the thumb, damage to the superficial radial nerve can result in sensory disturbance of both the dorsal and volar aspects of the thumb. In this instance, the volar basilar aspect of the thumb will be anesthetic, as will its usual "autonomous" dorsal region. On occasion, the volar aspect of the thumb can be anesthetic if the superficial radial also supplies this aspect of the thumb.

Surgery adjacent to the ulnar border of the flexor carpi radialis must be performed carefully in order to avoid injury to this sensory branch (Fig. 102). It is often best to identify this major branch before definitive surgery is performed in this region of the distal forearm and wrist (Fig. 101D). It is especially vulnerable during carpal tunnel releases and release of the flexor carpi radialis tunnel because of chronic localized tenosynovitis (Fig. 101A–C), tendon transfer procedures, the repair of lacerated wrist structures, and removal of soft tissue volar wrist lesions.

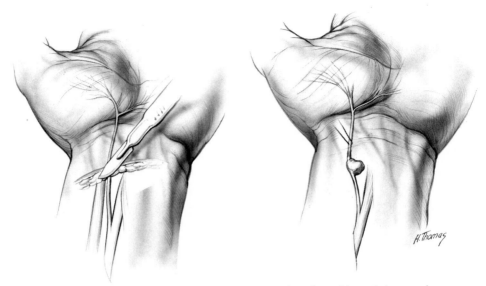

Figure 102.   The median palmar cutaneous nerve is vulnerable to injury and neuroma formation, especially when transverse incisions are utilized in the distal forearm on the radiovolar aspect. After its takeoff from the median nerve the median palmar cutaneous branch has a relatively superficial course just deep to the antebrachial fascia of the forearm on the medial side of the flexor carpi radialis tendon sheath.

Persistent pain after carpal tunnel release may be due not to incomplete release of the tunnel but rather to neuroma formation, either at the level of the wrist or in the surgical scar in the palm. It has been recommended that the surgical incision be located on the ulnar side of the axis of the ring finger, in the palm. The antebrachial fascia and the flexor retinaculum should be incised along this axis, or ulnar to this axis, in order to avoid injury to the terminal branches of the median palmar cutaneous nerve.[110]

Considering all the variations that can occur in the supply of the median palmar cutaneous nerve, to accurately place the palmar incision for carpal tunnel surgery, a local anesthetic block of this branch just proximal to the wrist on the medial border of the flexor carpi radialis will localize the ulnar border of its field of innervation in the palm. Thus, the skin incision for a specific patient could be accurately placed to avoid incisional neuroma. This is of particular value when managing a patient with a prior history of multiple neural compression lesions. These patients are prone to postoperative superficial neuroma formation. This should be remembered when treating a patient who has a prior history of this postoperative complication.

I have seen several cases in which the median nerve has been cut distal to the takeoff of the median palmar cutaneous nerve, and in which the proximal retraction of the median nerve has been limited by the intact median nerve. In addition this sensory branch may tether the median nerve to the radial side of the carpal tunnel following wrist trauma or Volkmann's ischemia (Fig. 100*A*).

Riche-Cannieu Anastomosis

Riche[92] and Cannieu,[16] in the last decade of the 19th century, independently described an anastomosis in the palm between the motor branches of the median and ulnar nerves. In recent years, Mannerfelt[68] has revived interest in this cross communication. He has demonstrated this variant in several of his dissections. An incidence as high as 77 per cent of hands has been reported.[40]

There are four basic patterns to this variation:

1. An anastomosis in the substance of the adductor pollicis between the median and ulnar nerves.

2. A communicating branch from the motor branch of the median nerve coursing anterior to the radial head of the flexor pollicis brevis and the ulnar component passing deep to the ulnar head of this muscle.

3. Anastomosis between the two motor nerves across the first lumbrical.

4. Anastomosis between the branch of the deep ulnar nerve to the adductor pollicis or flexor pollicis brevis and the median nerve digital branch to the thumb or index finger.

The exact role of this cross communication is unclear. Gehwolf[36] assumed it to be sensory. Foerster,[30] as a result of war-wound studies, and Harness and Sekeles,[40] as a result of anatomical dissections, concluded that the anastomosis is of the motor type.

OPERATIVE APPROACH TO THE MEDIAN NERVE

For exploration of any of the median nerve branches it is best to approach the nerve proximal and distal to the injury, identifying the median nerve and tracing it through the involved area. The skin incision can be S-shaped, with the horizontal component at the flexion crease. When a more extensive exposure is necessary for both nerve exploration and tendon surgery, the incision described by Littler,[63] which parallels the pronator teres in the proximal forearm, is of great value. It curves gently down the forearm into the hand, paralleling the wrist flexion crease (Fig. 103). In this incision the radial corner of the incision paralleling the lower border of the pronator teres should be of full thickness because on a few occasions this edge has shown some delay in healing.

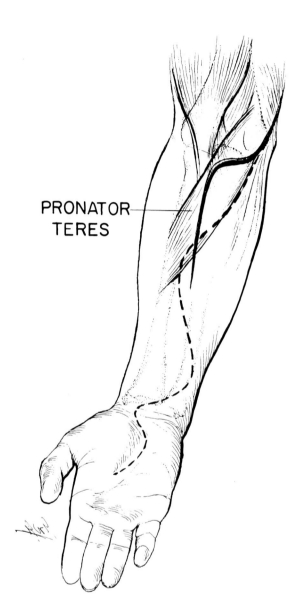

PRONATOR TERES

Figure 103.   The surgical incisions utilized to explore the median nerve and its branches. The dotted incision is for a more extensive exposure as recommended by Littler.

Once the skin has been incised and the fascia exposed and under-mined, the medial cutaneous nerves of the arm and forearm in the proximal third of the incision can be preserved (Fig. 123). The median nerve is identified proximal to the lacertus fibrosus and then traced distally. The safe side of the median nerve in the proximal forearm down to the level of the anterior interosseous branch is the radial side. The tendinous origin of the deep head of the pronator teres, frequently the offending structure in an anterior interosseous nerve syndrome, is iden-tified and detached (Fig. 104*A–C*). Special care must be taken to preserve the branches that innervate the medial epicondylar muscles when the ulnar side of the median nerve must be exposed in the antecubital fossa.

The median nerve in the proximal forearm dips through the prona-

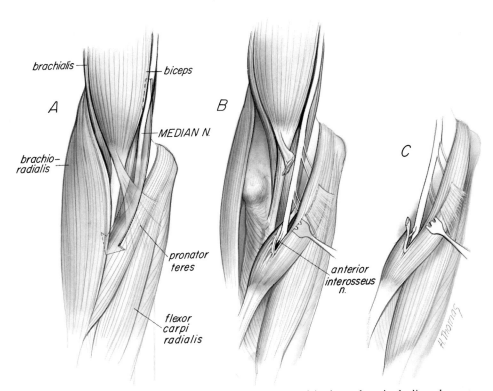

Figure 104.   *A*, For exposure of the median nerve and its branches, including the ante-rior interosseous, in the proximal third of the forearm, the median nerve is identified proximal to the lacertus fibrosus and is traced distally. *B*, The lacertus fibrosus is released, exposing the median nerve and its multiple branches. Proximally the branches arise from the medial side, while the anterior interosseous branch arises from the lateral side. *C*, The tendinous origin of the deep head of the pronator teres is released when tracing the anterior interosseous branch.

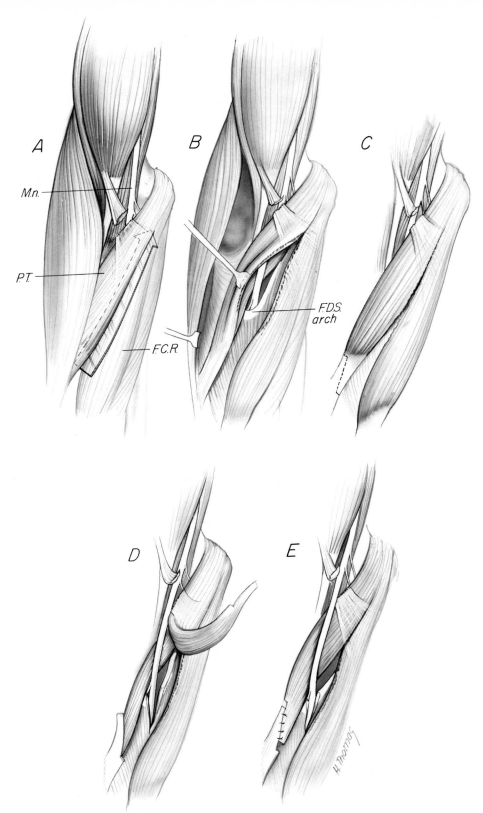

Figure 105.   *See legend on opposite page.*

tor heads in 82 per cent of limbs. At times the nerve may go deep to the ulnar head, and on occasion it may go through the humeral head. There are isolated reports of the median nerve passing anterior to the pronator teres. Because of these many variations, the best surgical approach when exploring the median nerve or any of its branches, such as the anterior interosseous nerve in the proximal half of the forearm, is to identify the median nerve proximal to the lacertus fibrosus and to trace it distally through the region of the pronator and the flexor superficialis arch.

The most convenient means of locating the median nerve under the pronator teres and the flexor carpi radialis is to identify the fascial plane between the flexor carpi radialis and the pronator teres more distally, and to develop this interval in a distal to proximal direction (Fig. 105C). The median nerve can be seen passing deep to the superficialis (Fig. 105B). For full exposure of the median nerve, the muscle of the pronator teres can be transected once the plane of the flexor carpi radialis and the pronator teres is well developed.

A more satisfying method of approaching the area is to lengthen the tendon of the pronator teres in a Z-plasty or tongue-shaped manner, thus exposing the median nerve and its branches. If the median nerve is to be passed anteriorly, the pronator teres can be passed deep to the median nerve, thus bringing the median nerve beneath the skin. The pronator teres is lengthened and resutured (Figs. 105C–E and 106).

This transposition anteriorly has been utilized when the entire median nerve required exploration or release, as in Volkmann's ischemic contracture of the forearm. In a patient with a pronator syndrome, after excision of the radial head, the median nerve was found to pass deep to both heads of the pronator teres. This rerouting of the median nerve by passing the entire pronator teres deep to the median nerve was found to be most effective in relieving the patient's symptoms. In addition, the 20- to 30-degree flexion contracture noted to be present at the elbow was corrected by lengthening the pronator teres. Most pronator

---

Figure 105.   To identify the median nerve through its course in the proximal forearm, the initial exposure as shown in Figure 104 is completed. The interval between the flexor carpi radialis (F.C.R.) and the pronator teres (P.T.) is developed, commencing the dissection in a distal to proximal direction (A). The common raphe between these two muscles is liberated. In the depth of the wound the flexor superficialis bridge (F.D.S. arch) crossing the median nerve (M.n.) is seen (B). The arch and any offending tendinous or fibrous structures impinging upon the median nerve can be released. D, Translocation of the median nerve anteriorly is accomplished by Z-plasty of the pronator teres. The flexor superficialis arch is incised. E, The pronator teres is passed posterior to the median nerve and resutured. It may be necessary to tease some of the branches from the median nerve trunk in order to allow for additional anterior mobilization of the nerve necessary to accomplish the translocation.

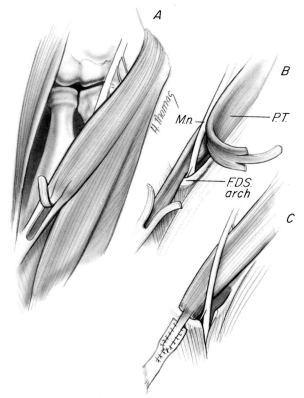

Figure 106. A tongue-shaped flap in the tendon of the pronator teres at its insertion can be utilized when performing an anterior translocation of the median nerve in the proximal forearm. Alternatively, a z-plasty of this tendon can be performed.

syndrome cases are relieved by releasing all offending tendinous and fibrous structures crossing the median nerve without anterior translocation of the nerve. This latter procedure is reserved for resistant cases, specific local anomalies, or scarred bed problems.

At the superficialis arch there are several small vessels crossing on the underside of the superficialis. These should be ligated when the flexor superficialis arch is split. The three branches of the median nerve to the superficialis are visualized and preserved. In the midportion of the arm, the accessory branch supplying the lower half of the flexor superficialis to the index finger is seen frequently and should be preserved. The one or two branches of the median palmar cutaneous are noted and are to be protected.

If one wishes to transpose an intact median nerve which is in a badly scarred bed, the median nerve should be brought to a subcutaneous position anterior to the pronator teres after that muscle has been lengthened. Resuture of the pronator teres deep to the nerve effectively brings the median nerve subcutaneous in the proximal third of the forearm. Where the median nerve passes deep to the flexor carpi radialis, and if the nerve is to be released from its scar bed without need for neurorrhaphy, then the flexor carpi radialis may be severed at its musculotendinous junction and then passed deep to the median nerve to be resutured. This gives the median nerve a completely subcutaneous course. However, if the median nerve is lacerated and length has to be gained, then the nerve can be brought back into the wound; its major branches are teased proximally from the main median nerve trunk to give more mobility to the nerve. The cut ends of the nerve are brought subcutaneously in the standard type repair when more than 4 inches of the median nerve have to be gained. Ordinarily this can be achieved by just flexing the wrist and elbow. On occasion, in cases requiring median neurorrhaphy in the midforearm, release of the tendinous deep head of the pronator teres alone allows for the extra mobilization in order to avoid the necessity of complete anterior translocation of the nerve.

BIBLIOGRAPHY

1. Ashby, B. S.: Hypertrophy of the Palmaris Longus. J. Bone Joint Surg., *46B*:230–232, 1964.
2. Assmus, H., Homer, J., and Martin, K.: Das Nervus-Interosseus-Anterior-Syndrom. Nervenarzt, *46*:659–661, 1975.
3. Baruch, A., and Hass, A.: Anomaly of the Median Nerve. J. Hand Surg., *2*:331–332, 1977.
4. Beaton, L. E., and Anson, B. J.: The Relation of the Median Nerve to the Pronator Teres Muscle. Anat. Rec., *75*:23–26, 1939.
5. Bell, G. E., Jr., and Goldner, J. L.: Compression Neuropathy of the Median Nerve. Southern Med. J., *49*:966–972, 1956.
6. Benini, A., and Tedeschi, N.: Die Schädigung des Nervus Interosseus Anterior (Kiloh-Nevin Syndrom). Schweiz. Med. Wschr., *104*:1695–1697, 1974.
7. Borchardt, M., and Wjasmenski, H.: Der Nervus Medianus. Beitr. f. Klin. Chir., *107*:553–582, 1917.
8. Brash, J. C.: Neuro-Vascular Hila of Limb Muscles. Edinburgh, E. and S. Livingstone, 1955.
9. Brooks, H. St. J.: Variations in the Nerve Supply of the Flexor Brevis Pollicis Muscle. J. Anat. Physiol., *20*:641–644, 1886.
10. Bucher, T. P. J.: Anterior Interosseous Nerve Syndrome. J. Bone Joint Surg., *54B*:555, 1972.
11. Buchthal, F., Rosenfalck, A., and Trojaborg, W.: Electrophysiological Findings in Entrapment of the Median Nerve at Wrist and Elbow. J. Neurol. Neurosurg. Psychiat., *37*:340–360, 1974.
12. Bugg, E. I., Jr., Coonrad, R. W., and Grim, K. B.: Giant-Cell Arteritis — An Acute Hand Syndrome. J. Bone Joint Surg., *45A*:1269–1272, 1963.
13. Butler, B., and Bigley, E.: Aberrant Index (First) Lumbrical Tendinous Origin Associated with Carpal-Tunnel Syndrome. A Case Report. J. Bone Joint Surg., *53A*:160–162, 1971.
14. Case, D. B.: A Pseudotumor of the Hand (An Abnormal Flexor Digitorum Sublimus). Postgrad. Med. J., *42*:574–575, 1966.
15. Carroll, R. E., and Green, D. P.: The Significance of the Palmar Cutaneous Nerve at the Wrist. Clin. Orthop., *83*:24–28, 1972.
16. Cannieu, J. M. A.: Recherches sur une Anastomose Entre la Branche Profunde du Cubitale et le Médian. Bull. Soc. d'Anat. Physiol. Bordeaux, *18*:339–340, 1897.
17. Cherington, M.: Proximal Pain in Carpal Tunnel Syndrome. Arch. Surg., *108*:69, 1974.
18. Crymble, B.: Brachial Neuralgia and the Carpal Tunnel Syndrome. Brit. Med. J., *3*:470–471, 1968.

19. Cseuz, K. A., Thomas, J. E., Lambert, E. H., Love, J. G., and Lipscomb, P. R.: Long-Term Results of Operation for Carpal Tunnel Syndrome. Mayo Clin. Proc., *41*:232–241, 1966.

20. Curtis, R. M., and Eversmann, W. W., Jr.: Internal Neurolysis as an Adjunct to the Treatment of the Carpal-Tunnel Syndrome. J. Bone Joint Surg., *55A*:733–740, 1973.

21. De Vecchis, L.: Su una Rara Sindrome Dissociata del Mediano all'Avambraccio (Sindrome di Kiloh-Nevin). Riv. Chir. Mano, *6*:110–115, 1968.

22. Dubreuil-Chambardel, L.: Variations des Artères du Membre Supérieur. Paris, Masson, 1926.

23. Eiken, O., Carstram, N., and Eddeland, A.: Anomalous Distal Branching of the Median Nerve. Scand. J. Plastic Reconstr. Surg., *5*:149–152, 1971.

24. Entin, M. A.: Carpal Tunnel Syndrome and Its Variants. Surg. Clin. N. Amer., *48*:1097–1112, 1968.

25. Fahey, J. J.: Fractures of the Elbow in Children. *In* Instructional Course Lectures, The American Academy of Orthopaedic Surgeons, Vol. XVII. St. Louis, The C. V. Mosby Co., 1960, pp. 13–46.

26. Farber, J. S., and Bryan, R. S.: The Anterior Interosseous Nerve Syndrome. J. Bone Joint Surg., *50A*:521–523, April 1968.

27. Fearn, C. B. d'A., and Goodfellow, J. W.: Anterior Interosseous Nerve Palsy. J. Bone Joint Surg., *47B*:91–93, Feb. 1965.

28. Ferner, H.: Ein abnormer Verhaluf des Nervus medianus vor dem M. pronator teres. Anat. Anz., *84*:151–156, 1937.

29. Finelli, P. F.: Anterior Interosseous Nerve Syndrome Following Cutdown Catheterization. Ann. Neurol., *1*:205–206, 1977.

30. Foerster, O.: Die Symptomatologie der Schussverletzungen der Peripheren Nerven. *In* M. Levandorosky (ed.): Handbuch der Neurologie. Berlin, Springer, 1929.

31. Furnas, D. W.: Muscle Tendon Variations in the Flexor Compartment of the Wrist. Plast. Reconstr. Surg., *36*:320–324, 1965.

32. Furusawa, S., Hara, T., Maehiro, S., Shiba, M., and Kondo, T.: Neuralgic Amyotrophy. Orthop. Surg. (Japan), *20*:1286–1296, 1969.

33. Gantzer, C. F. L.: De Musculorum Varietates. Thesis, Berlioni, J. F. Starckii, 1813.

34. Gardner, R. C.: Confirmed Case and Diagnosis of Pseudocarpal-Tunnel (Sublimis) Syndrome. New Eng. J. Med., *282*:858, 1970.

35. Gardner-Thorpe, C.: Anterior Interosseous Nerve Palsy: Spontaneous Recovery in Two Patients. J. Neurol., Neurosurg., Psychiat., *37*:1146–1150, 1974.

36. Gehwolf, S.: Weitere Fälle von Plexus bildung in der Hohlhand. Anat. Anz., *54*:435–440, 1921.

37. Gräper, L.: Eine sehr seltene Varietät des M. Flexor Digitorum Sublimis. Anat. Anz., *50*:80–94, 1917.

38. Graham, W. P., III: Variations of the Motor Branch of the Median Nerve at the Wrist. Plast. Reconstr. Surg., *51*:90–92, 1973.

39. Gruber, W.: Ueber die Verbindung des Nervus medianus mit dem Nervus ulnaris am Unterarme des Menschen und der Sängethiete. Arch. Anat. u. Physiol., *37*:501–522, 1870.

40. Harness, D., and Sekeles, E.: The Double Anastomotic Innervation of the Thenar Muscles. J. Anat., *109*:461–466, 1971.

41. Hartmann, H.: Note sur l'Anatomie des Nerfs de la Paume de la Main. Bull. Soc. Anat. Paris, *62*:860–864, 1887.

42. Hartmann, H.: Étude de Quelques Anastomoses Elliptiques des Nerfs du Membre Supérieur. Bull. Soc. Anat. Paris, *63*:151–164, 1888.

43. Hovelacque, A.: Anatomie des Nerfs Craniens et Rachidiens et du Système Grand Sympathique Chez L'Homme. Deuxième Partie, Paris, Gaston Doin et Cie, 1927, p. 451.

44. Huffmann, G., and Leven, B.: N. Interosseus Anterior-Syndrome. Bericht über 4 Eigene und 49 Fälle aus der Literatur. J. Neurol., *213*:317–326, 1976.

45. James, J. I. P.: A Case of Rupture of Flexor Tendons Secondary to Kienböck's Disease. J. Bone Joint Surg., *31B*:521–523, 1949.

46. Johnson, R. K., and Shrewbury, M. M.: Anatomical Course of the Thenar Branch of the Median Nerve — Usually in a Separate Tunnel Through the Transverse Carpal Ligament. J. Bone Joint Surg., *52A*:269–273, 1970.

47. Kaplan, E. B.: Correction of a Disabling Flexion Contraction of Thumb. Bull. Hosp. Joint Dis., *3*:51–54, 1942.

48. Kaplan, E. B.: Functional and Surgical Anatomy of the Hand. 2nd Ed., Philadelphia, J. B. Lippincott, 1965.

49. Kaplan, E. B.: Muscular and Tendinous Variations of the Flexor Superficialis of the Fifth Finger. Bull. Hosp. Joint Dis., *30*:59–67, 1969.

50. Kessler, I.: Unusual Distribution of the Median Nerve at the Wrist. A Case Report. Clin. Orthop., *67*:124–126, 1969.
51. Kiloh, L. G., and Nevin, S.: Isolated Neuritis of the Anterior Interosseous Nerve. Brit. Med. J., *1*:850–851, 1952.
52. Kojima, T., Harase, M., and Ietsune, T.: Pronator Syndrome, Report of Six Cases. Orthop. Surg. (Japan), *19*:1147–1148, 1968.
53. Kopell, H. P. and Thompson, W. A. L.: Pronator Syndrome. N. Engl. J. Med., *259*:713–715, 1958.
54. Krag, C.: Isolated Paralysis of the Flexor Pollicis Longus Muscle. An Unusual Variation of the Anterior Interosseous Nerve Syndrome. Case Report. Scand. J. Plast. Reconst. Surg., *8*:250–252, 1974.
55. Kummel, B. M., and Zazanis, G. A.: Shoulder Pain as the Presenting Complaint in Carpal Tunnel Syndrome. Clin. Orthop., *92*:227–230, 1973.
56. Lake, P. A.: Anterior Interosseous Nerve Syndrome. J. Neurosurg., *41*:306–309, 1974.
57. Lanz, U.: Variations of the Median Nerve at the Carpal Tunnel. Handchirurgie, 7:159–162, 1975.
58. Lanz, U.: Anatomical Variations of the Median Nerve in the Carpal Tunnel. J. Hand Surg., *2*:44–53, 1977.
59. Lejars, F.: L'Innervation de l'Eminence Thenar. Bull. Mem. Soc. Anat. Paris, t. IV, 5th Series, 433–437, 1890.
60. Lettin, A. W. F.: Carpal Tunnel Syndrome in Childhood. J. Bone Joint Surg., *47B*:556–559, 1965.
61. Linburg, R. M., and Albright, J. A.: An Anomalous Branch of the Median Nerve. A Case Report. J. Bone Joint Surg., *52A*:182–183, 1970.
62. Lipscomb, P. R., and Burelson, R. J.: Vascular and Neural Complications in Supracondylar Fractures in Children. J. Bone Joint Surg., *37A*:487–492, 1955.
63. Littler, J. W.: Principles of Reconstructive Surgery of the Hand. *In* Converse, J. M. (ed.): Reconstructive Plastic Surgery. Philadelphia, W. B. Saunders, 1964, p. 1635.
64. Luppino, T., Celli, L., and Montelone, M.: Paralisi Dissocita del Nervo Mediano all'Avambraccio da Compressione del Nervo Interosseo Anteriore. Chir. Organi Mov., *61*:89–94, 1972.
65. Maeda, K., Miura, T., Komada, T., and Chiba, A.: Anterior Interosseous Nerve Paralysis. Report of 13 Cases and Review of Japanese Literatures. Hand, *9*:165–171, 1977.
66. Mainland, D.: An Uncommon Abnormality of the Flexor Digitorum Sublimus Muscle. J. Anat., *62*:86–89, 1927.
67. Mangini, U.: Flexor Pollicis Longus Muscle. Its Morphology and Clinical Significance. J. Bone Joint Surg., *42A*:467–470, 1960.
68. Mannerfelt, L.: Studies on the Hand in Ulnar Nerve Paralysis. A Clinical-Experimental Investigation in Normal and Anomalous Innervation. Acta Orthop. Scand. Supplementum 87, 1966.
69. Mannerfelt, L.: Median Nerve Entrapment after Dislocation of the Elbow. J. Bone Joint Surg., *50B*:152–155, 1968.
70. Mannerfelt, L., and Hybbinette, C. H.: Important Anomaly of the Thenar Branch of the Median Nerve. Bull. Hosp. Joint Dis., *33*:15–21, 1972.
71. Martin, R.: Tal om Nervus allmanna Egenskaper i Mannsikans Kropp. Stockholm, Lars Salvius, 1763.
72. Matev, I.: A Radiological Sign of Entrapment of the Median Nerve in the Elbow Joint after Posterior Dislocation. J. Bone Joint Surg., *58B*:353–355, 1976.
73. Matsuzaki, A., Kobayashi, M., Mitsuyasu, M., Morooka, M., Honda, K., and Takeshima, Y.: Neuralgic Amyotrophy with the Feature of Palsy of the Anterior Interosseous Nerve. Orthop. Surg. (Japan), *20*:916–923, 1969.
74. Mauclaire, P. L.: Fôrme Nettement Digastrique de Plan Profound du Flechisseur Superficiel du Même Muscle Perforant le Nerf Médian. Des Dedoublements Réiproques des Nerfs, Artères, Veins et Muscles, Bull. Soc. Anat. Paris, 5th Series, *8*:75–81, 1894.
75. McLellan, D. L., and Swash, M.: Longitudinal Sliding of the Median Nerve During Movements of the Upper Limb. J. Neurol. Neurosurg. Psychiat., *39*:566–570, 1976.
76. Miller, R.: Observations upon the Arrangement of the Axillary Artery and Brachial Plexus, Am. J. Anat., *64*:143–163, 1939.
77. Mills, R. H., Mukherjee, K., and Bassett, I. B.: Anterior Interosseous Nerve Palsy. Brit. Med. J., *2*:555, 1969.
78. Morris, H. H., and Peters, B. H.: Pronator Syndrome: Clinical and Electrophysiological Features in Seven Cases. J. Neurol. Neurosurg. Psychiat., *39*:461–464, 1976.
79. Morrison, D. P., and Spinner, M.: Unpublished data.
80. Nakano, K. K., Lundergan, C., and Okihiro, M. M.: Anterior Interosseous Nerve Syndromes. Diagnostic Methods and Alternative Treatments. Arch. Neurol., *34*:477–480, 1977.

81. O'Brien, M. D., and Upton, A. R. M.: Anterior Interosseous Nerve Syndrome. A Case Report with Neurophysiological Investigation. J. Neurol. Neurosurg. Psychiat., *35*:531–536, 1972.

82. Ogden, J. A.: An Unusual Branch of the Median Nerve. J. Bone Joint Surg., *54A*:1779–1781, 1972.

83. Page, C. M.: An Operation for the Relief of Flexion-Contracture in the Forearm. J. Bone Joint Surg., *5*:233–234, 1923.

84. Papathanassiou, B. T.: A Variant of the Motor Branch of the Median Nerve in the Hand. J. Bone Joint Surg., *50B*:156–157, 1968.

85. Parsonage, M. J., and Turner, J. W. A.: Neuralgic Amyotrophy. The Shoulder-Girdle Syndrome. Lancet, *1*:973–978, 1948.

86. Passerini, D., and Vall, G.: Contributo alla Conoscenza della Sindrome del Nervo Interosseo Anteriore (Kiloh e Nevin). Riv. Pat. Nerv. Ment., *89*:1–11, 1968.

87. Phalen, G. S.: Reflections on 21 Years' Experience with the. Carpal-Tunnel Syndrome. J.A.M.A., *212*:1365–1367, 1970.

88. Pritchard, D. J., Linscheid, R. L., and Svien, H. J.: Intra-articular Median Nerve Entrapment with Dislocation of the Elbow. Clin. Orthop., *90*:100–103, 1973.

89. Rana, N. A., Kenwright, J., Taylor, R. G., and Rushworth, G.: Complete Lesion of the Median Nerve Associated with Dislocation of the Elbow Joint. Acta Orthop. Scand., *45*:365–369, 1974.

90. Ranschburg, P.: Über die Anastomosen der Nerven der oberen Extremität des Menschen mit Rücksicht auf ihre neurologische und Nerven chirurgische Bedentung. Neurol. Centralbl., *36*:521–534, 1917.

91. Reimann, A. F., Daseler, E. H., Anson, B. J., and Beaton, L. E.: The Palmaris Longus Muscle and Tendon. A Study of 1600 Extremities. Anat. Rec., *89*:495–505, 1944.

92. Riche, P.: Le Nerf Cubital et les Muscles de l'Eminence Thenar. Bull. Mem. Soc. Anat. Paris, *5*:251–252, 1897.

93. Rowntree, T.: Anomalous Innervation of the Hand Muscles. J. Bone Joint Surg., *51B*:505–510, 1949.

94. Schmidt, H., and Eiken, O.: The Anterior Interosseous Nerve Syndrome. Scand. J. Plast. Reconstr. Surg., *5*:53–56, 1971.

95. Schultz, R. J., Endler, P. M., and Huddleston, H. D.: Anomalous Median Nerve and an Anomalous Muscle Belly of the First Lumbrical Associated with Carpal-Tunnel Syndrome. J. Bone Joint Surg., *55A*:1744–1746, 1973.

96. Seyffarth, H.: Primary Myoses in the M. Pronator Teres as Cause of Lesion of the N. Medianus (The Pronator Syndrome). Acta Psychiat. et Neurol. Supplementum 74, 1951.

97. Shäfer, E. A., Symington, J., and Bryce, T. H. (Eds.): Quain's Anatomy Ed. 11, Vol. 3, Part 2. London, Longmanns, Green, and Co., 1909.

98. Sharrard, W. I. W.: Anterior Interosseous Neuritis. Report of a Case. J. Bone Joint Surg., *50B*:804–805, 1968.

99. Smith, B., and Herbst, B. A.: Anterior Interosseous Nerve Palsy. Arch. Neurol. (Chic.), *30*:330–331, 1974.

100. Solnitzky, O.: Pronator Syndrome: Compression Neuropathy of the Median Nerve at Level of Pronator Teres Muscle. Georgetown Med. Bull., *13*:232–238, 1960.

101. Spinner, M., and Schrieber, S. N.: The Anterior Interosseous-Nerve Paralysis as a Complication of Supracondylar Fractures in Children. J. Bone Joint Surg., *51A*:1584–1590, 1969.

102. Spinner, M.: The Anterior Interosseous-Nerve Syndrome. With Special Attention to its Variations. J. Bone Joint Surg., *52A*:84–94, 1970.

103. Spinner, M.: Cryptogenic Infraclavicular Brachial Plexus Neuritis. (Preliminary Report.) Bull. Hosp. Joint Dis., *37*:98–104, 1976.

104. Steiger, R. N., Larrick, R. B., and Meyer, T. L.: Median-Nerve Entrapment Following Elbow Dislocation in Children. J. Bone Joint Surg., *51A*:381–385, 1969.

105. Stellbrink, G.: Compression of the Palmar Branch of the Median Nerve by Atypical Palmaris Longus Muscle. Handchirurgie, *4*:155–157, 1972.

106. Stern, M. B., Rosner, L. J., and Blinderman, E. E.: Kiloh-Nevin Syndrome. Report of a Case and Review of the Literature. Clin. Orthop., *53*:95–98, 1967.

107. Sunderland, S.: The Innervation of the Flexor Digitorum Profundus and Lumbrical Muscles. Anat. Rec., *93*:317–321, 1945.

108. Sunderland, S.: The Intraneural Topography of the Radial, Median and Ulnar Nerves. Brain, *68*:243–299, 1945.

109. Sunderland, S.: Nerves and Nerve Injuries. Baltimore, The Williams and Wilkins Co., 1968.

110. Taleisnik, J.: The Palmar Cutaneous Branch of the Median Nerve and the Approach to the Carpal Tunnel. An Anatomical Study. J. Bone Joint Surg., *55A*:1212–1217, 1973.

111. Thomas, D. F.: Kiloh-Nevin Syndrome. J. Bone Joint Surg., *44B*:962, 1962.
112. Thomson, A.: Third Annual Report on the Committee of Collective Investigation of the Anatomical Society of Great Britain and Ireland for the Year 1891–1892. J. Anat. Physiol., *27*:183–194, 1893.
113. Tinel, J.: Nerve Wounds. New York, William Wood, 1918, pp. 183–185.
114. Vichare, N. A.: Spontaneous Paralysis of the Anterior Interosseous Nerve. J. Bone Joint Surg., *50B*:806–808, 1968.
115. Vichare, N. A.: Anomalous Muscle Belly of the Flexor Digitorum Superficialis. J. Bone Joint Surg., *52B*:757–759, 1970.
116. Warren, J. D.: Anterior Interosseous Nerve Palsy as a Complication of Forearm Fractures. J. Bone Joint Surg., *45B*:511–512, Aug. 1963.
117. Wesser, D. R., Calostypis, F., and Hoffman, S.: The Evolutionary Significance of an Aberrant Flexor Superficialis Muscle in the Human Palm. J. Bone Joint Surg., *51A*:396–398, 1969.
118. Wilson, S. A. K.: Neurology. London, Arnold, 1940, p. 329.
119. Winkelman, N. Z., and Spinner, M.: A Variant High Sensory Branch of the Median Nerve to the Third Web Space. Bull. Hosp. Joint Dis., *34*:161–166, 1973.
120. Woltman, H. W., and Kernohan, J. W.: Disease of Peripheral Nerves. *In* Baker, A. B. (ed.): Clinical Neurology. New York, Hoeber-Harper, 1955.

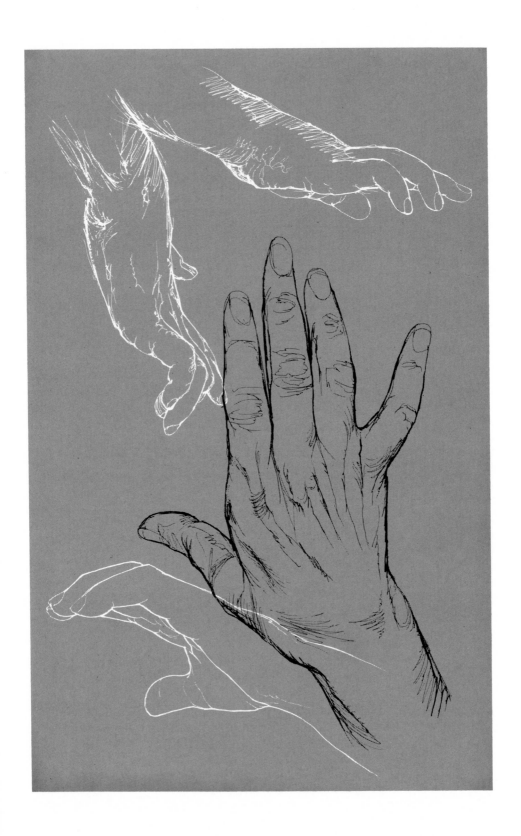

THE ULNAR NERVE

THE ULNAR NERVE

ANATOMY

The ulnar nerve runs a straight-line course through the forearm from the level of the medial epicondyle of the distal humerus to the pisiform-hamate groove in the carpus. It provides motor innervation to the flexor carpi ulnaris and the flexor profundus muscles of the ring and little fingers. It supplies sensory fibers to the dorsum of the hand on the ulnar side and to the dorsum of the fourth and fifth fingers, through the dorsal cutaneous nerve. This latter nerve arises on an average of 8 cm. proximal to the ulnar styloid. The motor branches to the flexor carpi ulnaris are usually two in number, one to the humeral and one to the ulnar head, although there may be one or two additional branches. They usually enter the muscle on its deep surface within the first 4 cm. distal to the medial epicondyle.

The flexor digitorum profundus branch arises from the ulnar nerve just distal to the branches of the flexor carpi ulnaris. It lies on the anterior surface of the flexor digitorum profundus and enters this muscle proximal to the motor supply to the adjacent flexor profundus muscles of the index and middle fingers, which is derived from the anterior interosseous nerve (median nerve). The motor supply to the ring and little fingers from the ulnar nerve usually enters the muscle of the flexor digitorum profundus about 6½ cm. distal to the medial epicondyle, while the anterior interosseous enters the flexor digitorum profundus 4 to 7 cm. more distally. The ulnar nerve, in relationship to the vessel, frames the forearm on the ulnar side, as does the superficial radial on the radial side. The ulnar artery when it approaches the ulnar nerve in the midforearm comes to lie on the radial side of the ulnar nerve. Similarly, the radial artery comes to lie on the inner or medial side of the superficial radial nerve. The ulnar nerve passes through a cubital tunnel in its course from the extensor surface behind the humerus to the forearm flexor surface. At the evel of the elbow joint, the nerve actually passes between the two heads of the flexor carpi ulnaris. There is a fascial connection between the two (Fig. 107A–C). Osborne[39, 40] and Vanderpool, Chalmers, Lamb and Whiston[59] have provided excellent descriptions of the finer anatomical details. The tunnel is elliptical and fibro-osseous. Laterally, it is bordered by the elbow joint and its transverse ligament, and medially by the aponeurosis between the two heads of the flexor carpi ulnaris.

At the distal end of the forearm, the ulnar artery and nerve enter the

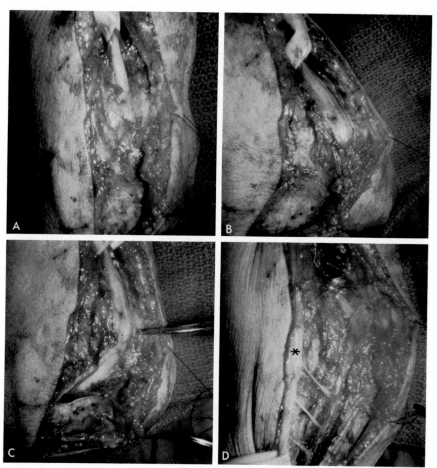

Figure 107.   Right elbow, *A*, The ulnar nerve has been identified proximal to the cubital tunnel. In extension the nerve is lax. *B*, In flexion the nerve becomes taut posterior to the medial epicondyle. *C*, The cubital tunnel has been opened. The two heads of the flexor carpi ulnaris—humeral and ulnar—are noted. The hemostat is at the most proximal portion of the cubital tunnel. *D*, The transposed ulnar nerve (*), the branches to the flexor carpi ulnaris and to the flexor digitorum profundus are visualized.

hand under a layer of thickened aponeurosis, originating as an extension of the flexor carpi ulnaris which attaches on the hook of the hamate. The area of passage under the aponeurotic expansion is called Guyon's tunnel.[13] It can be described as having a floor, a ceiling and two walls. The pisiform and the hamate with their ligamentous covering form the medial and lateral walls. The floor consists of the pisi-hamate ligament. The extent of the tunnel is 1½ cm. commencing from the distal flexion crease of the wrist under the origin of the abductor digiti quinti.

In the midforearm the ulnar nerve supplies its accompanying artery with a segmental sympathetic nerve. It is known as the nerve of Henle.[16] At the wrist sympathetic fibers arise from the distal ulnar nerve and supply the proximal ulnar portions of the superficial and deep vascular arches of the hand. The median nerve and the superficial radial nerve also give segmental supply to the superficial arch. The deep vascular arch is segmentally innervated by fibers from the ulnar nerve and the superficial radial nerve.

SIGNIFICANT ANATOMICAL VARIATIONS AND CLINICAL APPLICATIONS

Cubital tunnel.
Arcade of Struthers.
Anconeus epitrochlearis.
Ulnar nerve motor variants.
Sensory variations of the ulnar nerve.
Variations in the resting attitudes of the hand in ulnar nerve lesions.
Pseudoulnar claw hand.
Variations of Guyon's tunnel.

Cubital Tunnel

In the proximal forearm the most common cause for an idiopathic type of ulnar nerve paralysis is entrapment of the nerve at the cubital tunnel where the ulnar nerve enters the forearm posteriorly between the two heads of the flexor carpi ulnaris. A fascial connection is present between the two. The proximal edge may at times be thickened and may act as a compressing agent. Osborne[39, 40] and Vanderpool et al.[60] noted that with flexion the cubital tunnel decreases in volume and the aponeurosis becomes taut over the ulnar nerve. Rather than perform the anterior translocation procedures, Osborne and Vanderpool et al. have suggested that lysis or excision of the aponeurosis or even suture of the aponeurosis anterior to the ulnar nerve be performed to treat an entrapment in that location.

Numerous etiological factors can produce an ulnar nerve paralysis with localization at the elbow: idiopathic cubital tunnel syndrome, ganglion,[2] muscle anomaly (anconeus epitrochlearis), hypertrophic arthritis, non-union of an old fracture of the medial epicondyle, rheumatoid synovitis of the elbow joint,[8, 31] cubitus valgus, supracondyloid process,[10] snapping triceps,[43] and recurrent dislocation or subluxation of the ulnar nerve.[4] That external compression to the nerve at the cubital tunnel can be an additional factor has been emphasized by Wadsworth,[61] and the nerve is at risk when the forearm is pronated in bed, in an arm chair, or on the operating table.

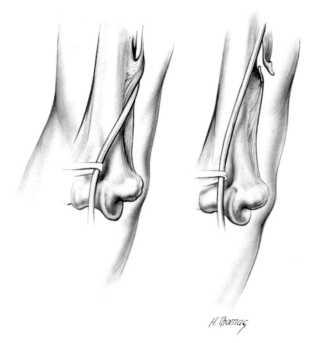

H. Thomas

Figure 108.   Approximately 8 cm. proximal to the medial epicondyle the ulnar nerve normally passes from anterior to the medial intermuscular septum to posterior to the septum. In anterior translocation of the ulnar nerve this arcade, if present, should be released.

In the past it has been recommended that ulnar neuritis secondary to localized symptoms referable to the elbow is best treated by translocation of the nerve anteriorly. Other authors have recommended excision of the medial epicondyle.[37] More recently, there appear to be good indications for simple excision of the fibrous arch between the humeral and the ulnar heads of the flexor carpi ulnaris.[9, 40, 60] The older method of anterior translocation of the nerve is best indicated for recurrent subluxations or dislocations of the ulnar nerve, advanced osteoarthritis posterior to the medial epicondyle, and cubitus valgus deformity.

With anterior translocation of the ulnar nerve there appear to be two major decisions, both based on the local anatomy, when considering the technique to be utilized: (1) going high enough and (2) translocating the nerve anteriorly in a subcutaneous plane or deep to the flexor pronator group of muscles (Learmonth procedure). Proximal to the elbow the ulnar nerve should be freed for at least 8 cm. from the medial epicondyle. Failure to do so may lead to a secondary ulnar neuritis at the level where the ulnar nerve passes from an anterior to a posterior plane in the arm (Fig. 108).

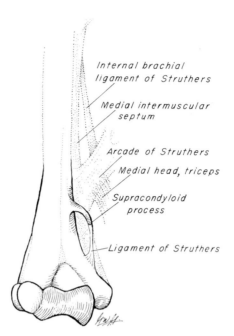

Internal brachial ligament of Struthers

Medial intermuscular septum

Arcade of Struthers

Medial head, triceps

Supracondyloid process

Ligament of Struthers

Figure 109.   A composite drawing adapted from Struthers (1848) original plate of the details of the supracondylar process in a right arm. The solid line section of the drawing demonstrates the ligament of Struthers arising from a supracondylar process and attaching to the junction of the medial epicondyle and the humeral metaphysis. The dotted portion, which is added to the original drawing, demonstrates the details of the level of the arcade. The supracondyloid process and the ligament of Struthers are anterior to the medial intermuscular septum, while the internal brachial ligament is posterior to it. (From Spinner, M., and Kaplan, E. B.: The Relationship of the Ulnar Nerve to the Medial Intermuscular Septum in the Arm and Its Clinical Significance. Hand, 8:239–242, 1976.)

Arcade of Struthers

This arcade was first described by Struthers[50, 51] in 1854. It is unrelated to the ligament he described in association with a supracondylar process[49] and which also bears his name (Fig. 109). The ligament of Struthers and the supracondylar process are found in only 1 per cent of all upper extremities. In an anatomical study of 20 limbs, we found the arcade (Fig. 110) to be present in 14 specimens (70 per cent).[20]

When the arm is in the anatomical position the roof of the arcade faces medially. It is formed by a thickening of the deep investing fascia of the distal part of the arm, by superficial muscular fibers of the medial head of the triceps, and by attachments of the internal brachial ligament. The internal brachial ligament can be traced back to its origin from the region of the coracobrachialis tendon. Its anterior border is the medial

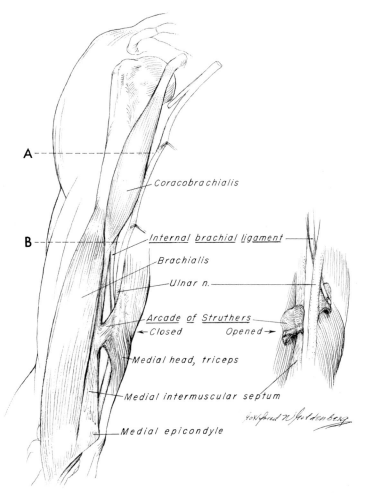

Figure 110.   Composite drawing of the arcade of Struthers and the internal brachial ligament. The ulnar nerve has been retracted to demonstrate the passage of the internal brachial ligament. *Insert:* The arcade has been opened. The course of the internal brachial ligament within the arcade is demonstrated. (From Spinner, M., and Kaplan, E. B.: The Relationship of the Ulnar Nerve to the Medial Intermuscular Septum in the Arm and Its Clinical Significance. Hand, *8:*239–242, 1976).

intermuscular septum. Laterally, the arcade is formed by the medial aspect of the humerus covered by deep muscular fibers of the medial head of the triceps.

The examiner should suspect the presence of this arcade when, on tracing the ulnar nerve proximally from the medial epicondyle, muscle fibers of the medial head of the triceps are seen crossing obliquely, superficial to the nerve (Figs. 111*A* and *B* and 112). When no muscular fibers cross the ulnar nerve 5 to 7 cm. proximal to the medial epicondyle, the arcade is not present (Fig. 111*C*).

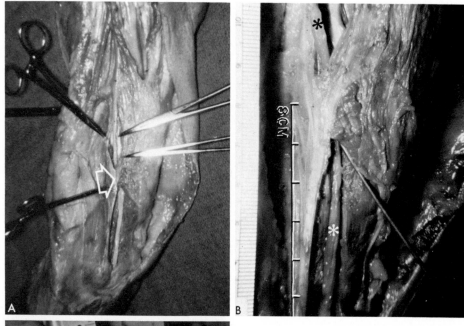

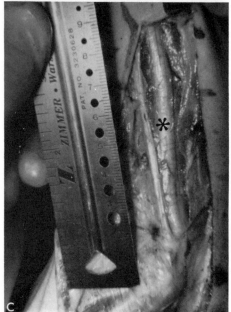

Figure 111. *A*, Right arm cadaver dissection demonstrates the ulnar nerve passing deep to the medial intermuscular septum at the level of the arcade of Struthers (arrow). *B*, Closeup view of the distal medial aspect of this arm. The probe is under the arcade. Note the muscular fibers of the superficial portion of the medial head of the triceps crossing the ulnar nerve (asterisks) in presence of the arcade of Struthers. *C*, At surgery in this right arm no arcade was found, and there were no muscular fibers crossing the ulnar nerve (asterisk).

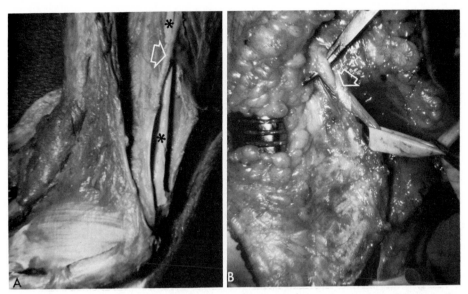

Figure 112.   *A*, Right cadaver arm with the arcade of Struthers (arrow) and with superficial muscular fibers of the medial head of the triceps crossing the ulnar nerve (asterisk). *B*, At surgery a right arm with recurrent ulnar nerve symptoms in which the arcade (arrow), 8 cm. proximal to the medial epicondyle, had not been released when the nerve was translocated anteriorly by the initial surgeon.

At the elbow three mechanical factors can affect this nerve — compression, stretch, and friction. They all can play a part in the production of the neural dysfunction (Fig. 113). Compression can occur above the elbow at the arcade, at the level of the medial epicondylar groove, or distally as the nerve passes between the ulnar and humeral heads of the flexor carpi ulnaris. It has been demonstrated that during elbow flexion the nerve stretches and elongates approximately 4.7 mm.[1] In addition, during flexion the medial head of the triceps was found to push the ulnar nerve anteromedially 0.73 cm. When there is fixation of the nerve a traction neuritis can develop. A friction neuritis can be caused by repeated movement and rubbing of the nerve against callus or irregularities of the posterior aspect of the distal humerus. An arcade of Struthers, when present, may be a contributing factor in the pathomechanics associated with the production of an ulnar nerve paralysis.

When completing the ulnar nerve translocation distally, the nerve should be in a straight line without knuckling as it passes down the forearm (Fig. 114C). The nerve is allowed to pass subcutaneously (Fig. 114) or is rerouted deep to the flexor–pronator group of muscles (Fig. 115). This latter technique was described by Sir James Learmonth in 1942.[29] For either procedure it is best to expose the nerve through a medial incision, passing posterior to the medial epicondyle and allowing

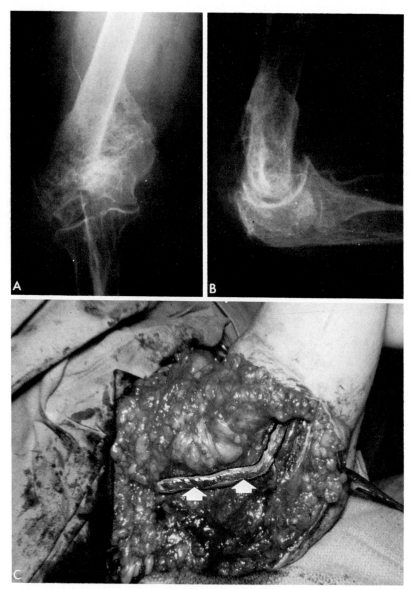

Figure 113.   *A,* Anteroposterior roentgenogram of the right elbow with a cubitus varus deformity of a supracondylar fracture of the humerus in a 68-year-old female. *B,* The lateral roentgenogram reveals considerable callus and irregularity of the bone posteriorly in the course of the ulnar nerve. *C,* Because of persistent and severe neuritic pain, the ulnar nerve was explored and found to be markedly thickened (arrows) at the time of the anterior translocation. The thickening of the nerve was probably due to all three mechanical factors — compression, stretch and friction.

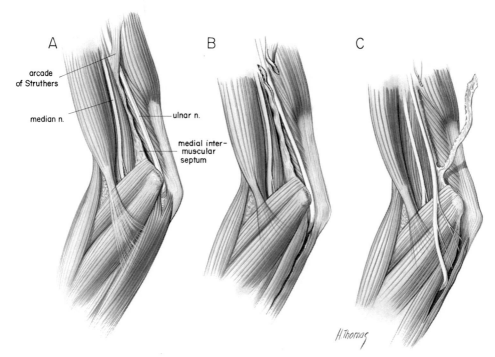

A

arcade
of Struthers

median n.

ulnar n.

medial inter-
muscular
septum

B

C

H. Thomas

Figure 114. *A,* When the ulnar nerve is translocated anteriorly, the ulnar nerve, the medial intermuscular septum, and the arcade of Struthers are exposed. *B,* The arcade is released. *C,* The medial intermuscular septum is removed and the ulnar nerve is dissected distally so that when it is transferred subcutaneously and anteriorly, distal kinking should be prevented. It should be noted that the ulnar nerve is now anterior throughout its course in the arm.

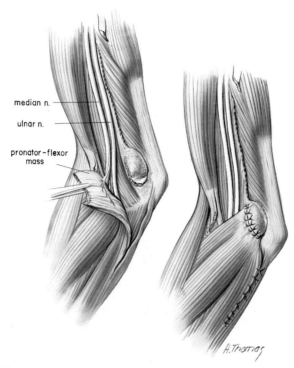

median n.

ulnar n.

pronator-flexor
mass

H.Thomas

Figure 115.   With the Learmonth procedure the ulnar nerve is translocated anteriorly and deep to the flexor-pronator muscles. The flexor-pronator muscles are resutured to their origin. Proximally, the ulnar nerve is liberated to above 8 cm. proximal to the medial epicondyle, the medial intermuscular septum is excised, and the arcade of Struthers is released. When the ulnar nerve is translocated deep to the flexor-pronator muscles it is brought adjacent to the medial nerve and its surrounding fat. Care is taken not to injure the anterior interosseous branch of the median nerve, which arises in this region.

for preservation of the medial cutaneous nerves of the arm and forearm (Fig. 116). Failure to preserve these skin nerves can result in painful postoperative neuromata.

It is not wise to put the translocated ulnar nerve in a groove in the flexor–pronator group of muscles because a resultant postoperative traction neuritis is a frequent complication of this technique (Fig. 117*A* and *B*). The disorder is caused by the adherent, longitudinally oriented, aponeurotic, fibrous attachments of the pronator teres, flexor carpi radialis, and flexor carpi ulnaris. The pain derived from this procedure can be lessened by liberating the nerve in its muscular-aponeurotic bed and converting the operation technically to the Learmonth type (Fig. 117*C*).

Anconeus Epitrochlearis

The anconeus epitrochlearis[30] is an anomalous muscle that arises from the medial border of the olecranon and adjacent triceps tendon and

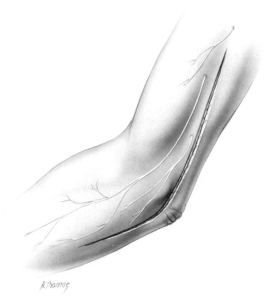

Figure 116.   The skin incision utilized when translocating the ulnar nerve.

inserts into the medial epicondyle. It crosses the ulnar nerve posterior to the cubital tunnel. It is an auxiliary extension of the medial portion of the triceps. When present it forms part of the cubital tunnel, reinforcing the aponeurosis of the two heads of origin of the flexor carpi ulnaris. It has been found to be a factor in producing ulnar compressive neuritis posterior to the elbow. Excision of the mass without translocation of the nerve has relieved symptoms when it was the sole factor in the pathogenesis. If there is osteoarthritis of the medial epicondyle, translocation of the ulnar nerve is the procedure of choice.

Ulnar Motor Nerve Variants

Variations occur in the manner in which the nerves branch in the proximal forearm. Instead of two or three branches to the flexor carpi ulnaris there may be as many as five, and there may be two branches to the flexor digitorum profundus. In isolated case reports the flexor carpi ulnaris was found to have a motor branch from the median nerve. In this instance weak action of this muscle may be observed when a complete high ulnar lesion is present.

Within the muscle belly of the flexor profundus major variations of its innervation occur. Here, the branch or branches of the ulnar nerve may innervate more of the profundus muscle supplying completely or partially the long finger as well as the ring and little fingers. Initially

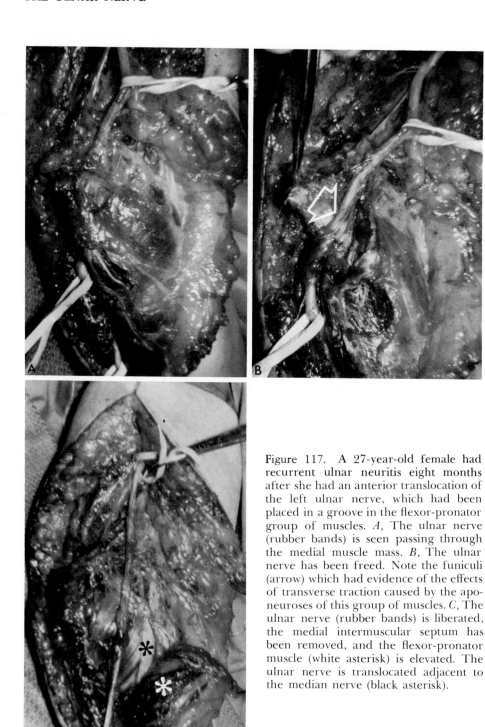

Figure 117. A 27-year-old female had recurrent ulnar neuritis eight months after she had an anterior translocation of the left ulnar nerve, which had been placed in a groove in the flexor-pronator group of muscles. *A*, The ulnar nerve (rubber bands) is seen passing through the medial muscle mass. *B*, The ulnar nerve has been freed. Note the funiculi (arrow) which had evidence of the effects of transverse traction caused by the aponeuroses of this group of muscles. *C*, The ulnar nerve (rubber bands) is liberated, the medial intermuscular septum has been removed, and the flexor-pronator muscle (white asterisk) is elevated. The ulnar nerve is translocated adjacent to the median nerve (black asterisk).

Sunderland[52] had stated that the profundus to the index finger was the only one that was always supplied by the anterior interosseous nerve (median), but later he added one case in which the ulnar nerve supplied even the profundus to the index finger.[53] It is through this motor branch of the ulnar nerve that the variations occur and the overlap into the sphere innervated by the median nerve through the anterior interosseous nerve takes place.

Likewise, when an "all median nerve hand" does occur the anterior interosseous nerve may supply more and more of the muscular bellies of the flexor digitorum profundus, and it is possible, as in the "all median hand," for the anterior interosseous to supply the entire flexor digitorum profundus. The flexor carpi ulnaris may at times receive additional motor supply from the ulnar nerve in the midforearm. This accessory branch is inconstant.

The Riche-Cannieu[3, 42] anastomosis in the palm between the deep branch of the ulnar nerve and the motor branch of the median nerve is another of the potential crossing neural pathways. There is some question regarding its incidence and whether this communication is sensory or motor.[34] In the distal forearm a crossing of fibers from the ulnar nerve to the median nerve occurs with less frequency than in the opposite direction (Martin-Gruber anastomosis). These cross communications help explain unexpected function in a hand when a major nerve is severed.

At the level of the wrist, in the region of the hypothenar eminence, variations of the ulnar nerve and its terminal branches can occur. The deep motor branch of the ulnar nerve, which usually passes distal to the hook of the hamate, can be split, with one portion passing radially to the hook and the other medially. These two branches then rejoin distally.[26, 27] A partial or complete motor paralysis of the intrinsic muscles of the hand can develop spontaneously. An anomalous terminal branch of the ulnar nerve has been observed at the distal end of Guyon's tunnel, which joined the digital sensory branch to the medial aspect of the little finger.[5] A combined motor and partial sensory paralysis can be a resultant finding with this anatomical arrangement. Shea and McClain[46] observed three clinical patterns of entrapment lesions of the ulnar nerve at the wrist — combined motor and sensory loss, sensory loss, and motor loss. The anatomical variants may lead to a variety of clinical manifestations, all dependent on the anatomical arrangement, which will be aggravated by local pathological processes, such as ulnar artery thrombosis,[6] ganglia,[2, 59] anomalous muscles,[18, 45, 47, 55, 57, 59, 62] fibrotic arches,[15, 36, 59] and trauma.

It must be remembered that, in addition to local pathology of the deep branch of the ulnar nerve, isolated atrophy of the intrinsic muscles can be caused by foramen magnum meningioma[33] and anterior horn cell disease.

Sensory Variations of the Ulnar Nerve

The dorsal cutaneous nerve varies in the way it branches from the ulnar nerve. Six to 8 cm. proximal to the wrist joint is the average point of take-off but it can vary significantly from this. This sensory branch can arise from the ulnar nerve as far proximal as the elbow and travel subcutaneously the entire length of the forearm.[41] One interesting variation was described by Dr. Emanuel B. Kaplan,[21] in which an entire loop was formed about the pisiform between the ulnar nerve and a branch from the dorsal cutaneous nerve. This branch of the dorsal cutaneous nerve appeared to add additional fibers to the ulnar digital nerve of the fifth finger, just as if some of the volar sensory fibers to the ulnar side of the fifth finger had gone with the dorsal cutaneous ulnar nerve and then had to reroute back to the volar area of the fifth finger.

Learmonth[28] has reported complete absence of the ulnar dorsal cutaneous nerve, with the superficial radial nerve increasing its region of distribution to include the usual ulnar sensory area of the dorsum of the hand and fingers. In this instance injury to, or a lesion of, the ulnar nerve at the elbow would not produce sensory loss of the dorsum of the hand but would present with sensory findings similar to those of a low ulnar nerve lesion. It should be suspected if electromyographic localization is at the elbow when clinical findings suggest the wrist. The presence of this variation can be confirmed by local block anesthesia of the superficial radial nerve. A similar diagnostic problem occurs when the dorsal branch of the musculocutaneous nerve takes over the sensory supply of the dorsoulnar area of the hand. It too can be recognized by electromyographic studies in conjunction with a local block of the musculocutaneous nerve.

The dorsoulnar aspect of the hand is usually innervated by the dorsal cutaneous branch of the ulnar nerve, but it can be supplied by the superficial radial nerve, the dorsal division of the musculocutaneous nerve, or the posterior cutaneous nerve of the forearm (Fig. 118D). The ulnar nerve usually innervates the volar aspect of the medial 1½ digits. This pattern is quite variable, as the area of ulnar innervation can extend to include the medial 2, 2½, or 3 digits (Fig. 118A C). In some cases only the volar aspect of the little finger is innervated by the ulnar nerve. The ulnar supply to the fourth web space (i.e., to the ulnar side of the ring finger and the radial side of the little finger), instead of arising in its usual location at the distal end of Guyon's tunnel, has been observed to arise in the midforearm and travel an aberrant course superficial to the transverse carpal ligament and the palmar aponeurosis.[58] If present, it can be vulnerable to injury during carpal tunnel surgery and other routine hand surgical procedures in this region.

The dorsal cutaneous branch of the ulnar nerve can develop a

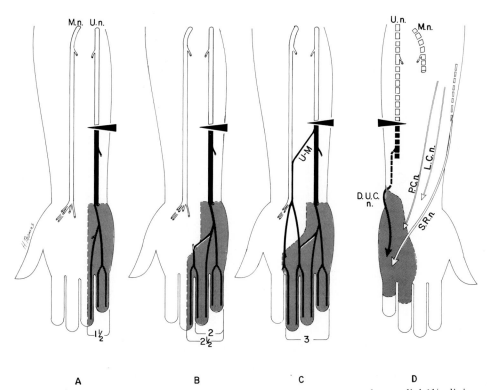

Figure 118.   The typical sensory distribution of the ulnar nerve to the medial 1½ digits, *A* can be increased to the adjacent digits by neural communications in the palm (*B*) and in the forearm (*C*). *D*, The superficial radial nerve (S.R.n.) can supply the dorsoulnar aspect of the hand, which is usually innervated by the dorsal ulnar cutaneous nerve (D.U.C.n.). The posterior cutaneous nerve of the forearm (P.C.n.) and the lateral cutaneous nerve of the forearm (L.C.n.) can also supply some of the dorsoulnar aspect of the hand. (From Omer, G., and Spinner, M.[12]: Peripheral Nerve Testing and Suture Techniques. *In* American Academy of Orthopedic Surgeons Instructional Course Lectures, Vol. 24. St. Louis, C. V. Mosby, 1975, pp. 122–143.)

troublesome neuroma, especially with avulsion injuries of the dorsum of the hand. The neuroma can adhere to the traumatized extensor tendon of the little finger and produces pain by active flexion and extension of the digit (Fig. 119).

The dorsal cutaneous nerve can be compressed by external pressure in people who write with their left hand. Often, these people write with the ulnar border of the wrist against the firm writing surface. If the dorsal cutaneous branch of the ulnar nerve passes from its volar position to the dorsum of the hand over the bony prominence of the distal ulna, then the external compression can cause symptoms of pain in the wrist and numbness of the dorsoulnar aspect of the hand to develop. The patient's symptoms can be relieved by resting the hand, by padding the

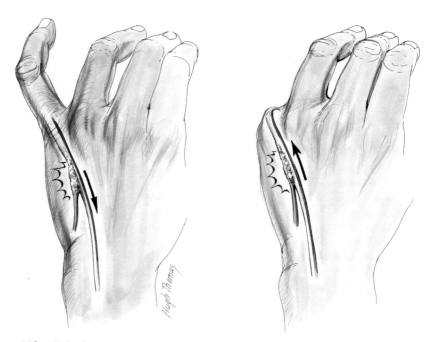

Figure 119.   Pain due to a neuroma of the dorsal cutaneous branch of the ulnar nerve is not an uncommon finding, especially if the neuroma becomes adherent to the extensor tendon of the little finger. Pain is produced with active flexion and extension of the digit.

ulnar aspect of the wrist, and by changing the writing pattern and its intensity. The symptoms will recur if the writing pattern is not changed. Surgical intervention is not recommended.

The ulnar palmar cutaneous nerve is not a constant branch as is its counterpart, the median palmar cutaneous nerve. When present, it arises at variable levels from the ulnar nerve in the lower half of the forearm. Neuromata of this nerve have not been recognized as a problem as they are with the median palmar cutaneous nerve, where injuries frequently result in marked symptomatology. I have seen one patient in whom I suspected this branch to have been cut, because the level of the skin laceration was within 2 cm. of the distal volar crease on the ulnar side. There was dry skin in a 4 × 3 cm. area at the base of the hypothenar eminence. The ring and little fingers had normal sensation, as did the dorsum of the hand and fingers. There was full motor function in the hand.

Variations in the Resting Attitudes of the Hand in Ulnar Nerve Lesions

When an ulnar lesion exists, the attitude of the hand depends on whether the lesion is high or low. The high ulnar lesion, occurring anywhere in the arm down to the level of the motor branches to the long extrinsic flexors of the ring and fifth fingers, results in an attitude quite different from that produced by a low lesion. Excluding anatomical variants of the ulnar nerve, one cannot distinguish the level of a motor nerve lesion solely by motor examination and/or by the resting attitude of the hand. Careful sensory examination and segmental electroneuro-myographic methods are essential to clarify the precise level of the lesion. The only difference in the lesion between the wrist and the midforearm is the sensory changes that occur with the lesion proximal to the takeoff of the dorsal cutaneous nerve. A low ulnar hand with a sensory loss on the dorsum of the ulnar aspect of the hand indicates a lesion in the fore-arm proximal to the dorsal cutaneous nerve, but distal to the motor branches to the flexor digitorum profundus of the ring and little fingers. The full-blown low lesion with sensory loss only at the volar aspect of the ulnar half of the ring and the entire fifth finger as well as a small portion of the distal area of the dorsum of the fifth finger has the motor appear-ance of a claw of the fourth and fifth fingers (Fig. 120 C–E), while a lesion proximal to the motor branch of the flexor profundus of the little and ring fingers does not yield a claw finger. On clinical examination there is evidence that the function of the profundus muscle of the fourth and fifth fingers is absent. In certain cases, when the ulnar nerve supplies the second lumbrical (to the long finger), the long finger may also be clawed in a low ulnar lesion (Figs. 120 F and 121 A). If in a low ulnar nerve lesion the lumbrical of the long finger is innervated by the median nerve, there is clawing of the little finger only (Fig. 121B).

A high ulnar nerve lesion usually presents with a normal appearing hand, but it can also be seen with a claw hand (Fig. 122). Thus, the same high level ulnar nerve lesion can reveal either a "normal" appearing hand or a claw hand. With a high ulnar nerve lesion a claw hand occurs if the anterior interosseous branch of the median nerve supplies the flexor profundus to all the digits.

It is essential to preserve the nerve to the flexor digitorum profun-dus in the proximal forearm, because if it is damaged the hand is converted into a high ulnar lesion. I have seen this occur in a patient who had a complete lower ulnar lesion when the nerve was mobilized to gain length and the proximal branch had been sacrificed, resulting in a loss of function of the fourth and fifth fingers. This complicated the reconstruc-tion; instead of just restoring intrinsic muscle function, it was necessary to re-establish the extrinsic flexor power of the fourth and fifth fingers as well. These branches of the ulnar nerve are susceptible to damage in muscle slide procedures (Fig. 123) and during translocation of the ulnar nerve for a traumatic ulnar neuritis arising behind the elbow (Fig. 107D).

A low ulnar nerve injury can be mistaken for a high motor nerve

Text continued on page 252

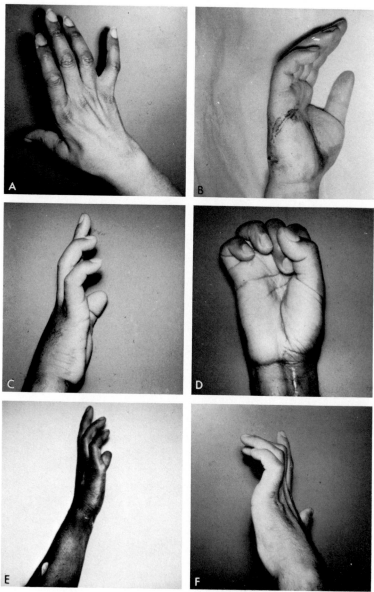

Figure 120.   *A*, Inability to adduct the fifth finger is a frequent residue of ulnar nerve injury. Note the commonly observed atrophy of the first dorsal interosseous muscle. *B*, The right hand has been shot. The powder wound of the bullet entrance is between the thenar and hypothenar eminence. The exit wound is seen adjacent to the fifth meta-carpal. Both the carpal and Guyon's tunnel presented with compressive symptomatology. *C* and *D*, Ulnar claw but with additional difficulty with residual extension contracture of the metacarpophalangeal joints of the fourth and fifth fingers. In *D* the ring finger and little finger could not be flexed into the palm when the patient attempted to make a fist. *E*, Bullet wound of the forearm produced this ulnar claw hand. *F*, A low ulnar nerve lesion which involves not only the ring and little fingers but the long finger as well.

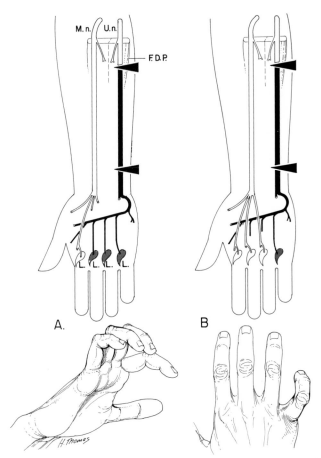

Figure 121.   *A*, A complete ulnar nerve lesion results in a three-finger clawhand when the lumbrical to the long finger is innervated by the ulnar nerve. *B*, Claw deformity of the little finger only occurs with a complete low ulnar lesion when the ring finger lumbrical is innervated by the median nerve. (From Omer, G., and Spinner, M.: Peripheral Nerve Testing and Suture Techniques. *In* American Academy of Orthopedic Surgeons Instructional Course Lectures, Vol. 24, St. Louis, C. V. Mosby, 1975, pp. 122–143.)

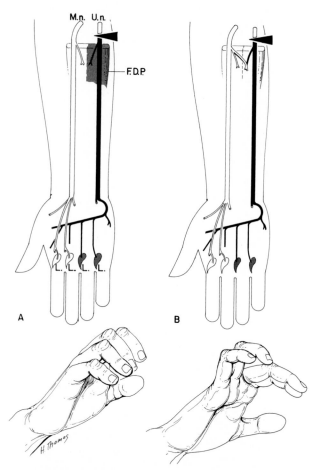

Figure 122. *A,* A complete high ulnar nerve lesion is usually observed without digital claw deformity. *B,* However, complete high ulnar nerve lesions produce a clawed hand when the intact median nerve supplies the flexor digitorum profundus to the ring finger and little finger. (From Omer, G., and Spinner, M.: Peripheral Nerve Testing and Suture Techniques. *In* American Academy of Orthopedic Surgeons Instructional Course Lectures, Vol. 24, St. Louis, C. V. Mosby, 1975, pp. 122–143.)

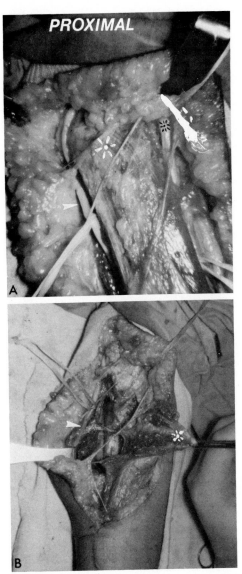

Figure 123.   Muscle slide procedure in the left forearm. *A,* Both the ulnar nerve (arrow) and median nerve (black *) are identified as well as the medial cutaneous nerves of the forearm and arm. *B,* The medial pronator-flexor group of muscles (white *) is elevated from the medial epicondyle and the proximal forearm.

injury when, in addition to the nerve injury, the flexor profundus muscles of the ring and little fingers are cut. The level of the laceration at the wrist or distal forearm can help clarify this problem.

Even with a complete high or low ulnar nerve lesion, the hand may not have any obvious loss of function. The resting attitude of the hand can be normal in appearance. This can occur when there are variant neural connections between the median and ulnar nerves in the forearm and hand (Fig. 124).

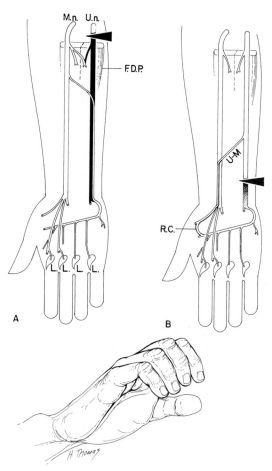

Figure 124. *A,* Here, a high ulnar nerve lesion has a normal attitude even though the flexor profundus muscles of the index, long, ring, and little fingers are innervated by the anterior interosseous branch of the median nerve because the intrinsic muscles are also innervated by the anomalous Martin-Gruber communication. *B,* Similarly, a complete low ulnar nerve lesion can also present with a normal-appearing hand when both an ulnar to median nerve (U-M) and a Riche–Cannieu (R.C.) communication are present (From Omer, G., and Spinner, M.: Peripheral Nerve Testing and Suture Techniques. *In* American Academy of Orthopedic Surgeons Instructional Course Lectures, Vol. 24, St. Louis, C. V. Mosby, 1975, pp. 122–124.)

Partial injury to the ulnar nerve in the forearm and just proximal to the wrist can be confusing if the possibility of a partial lesion is not considered, for such a lesion may produce symptoms of motor or sensory involvement alone. In the rare occasion when the median nerve supplies all the intrinsics ("the all median hand"), a complete nerve lesion may be represented only by a loss of sensation in the fifth finger and part of the ring finger. In certain puncture injuries produced by butcher knives or stilettos, I have seen just a portion of the ulnar nerve (either sensory or motor) divided (Fig. 125).

Derangements of the distal radioulnar joint may be associated with ulnar nerve paresis or paralysis.[11] Locked anterior fracture-dislocation of

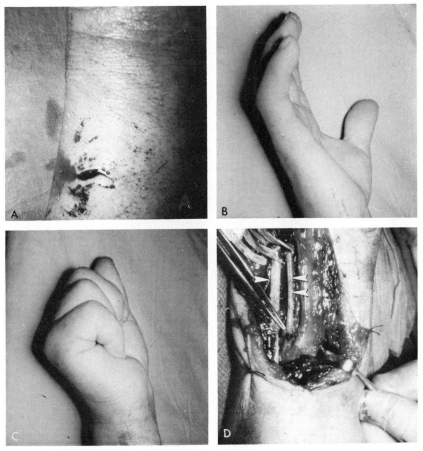

Figure 125.   *A*, A butcher's knife slipped, producing a small entrance wound. The skin was tense and there was considerable subfascial bleeding. *B*, An ulnar claw hand was present. *C*, The fingers flex well. *D*, The operative field demonstrates the damage to the ulnar nerve (one arrow) and to the adjacent ulnar artery (two arrows). The profuse bleeding in the fascial compartment of the forearm required prompt surgical treatment which included fascicular repair and fasciotomy.

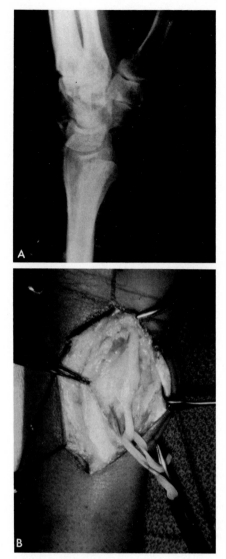

Figure 126.   *A*, The ulnar styloid of the left wrist is fractured. There is a locked anterior dislocation of the distal radioulnar joint. *B*, The ulnar nerve is compressed on the anteriorly displaced distal ulnar head.

Figure 127.   *A*, Note the deformity of this left wrist due to a compound fracture of the wrist with both median and ulnar nerve involvement. *B*, Anteroposterior roentgenogram reveals comminuted fracture at the distal end of the radius and ulnar styloid. *C*, The median nerve (asterisk) is traced through the carpal tunnel. The ulnar nerve (arrow) was found to dip into the distal radioulnar joint. *D*, Upon reduction the traumatized ulnar

Illustration continued on opposite page

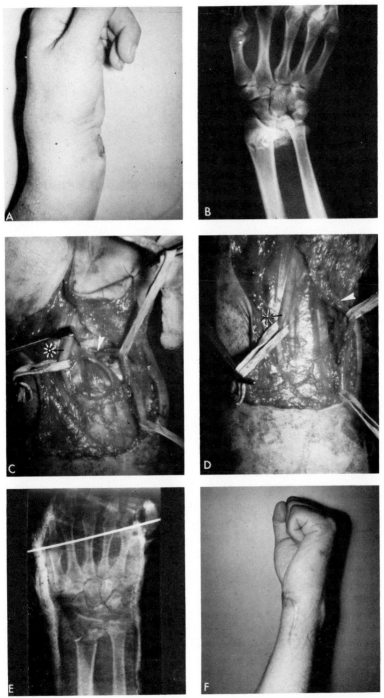

nerve (arrow) and the median nerve (asterisk) were restored to their usual course. *E*, Reduction of the fracture was maintained in a long-arm cast with one small Steinmann pin through the second and third metacarpals and a second through the olecranon. *F*, The patient regained full sensation and full range of movement of the fingers by the end of 6 months.

the distal ulna (Fig. 126), Colles fracture, pisiform or hamate fracture, intercarpal dislocations, and even fractures of the basis of the metacarpals may present with this neural complication.[17] In one case of a compound and severely comminuted fracture of the distal radius and ulna, the ulnar nerve was found to be trapped in the distal radioulnar joint (Fig. 127).

Pseudoulnar Claw Hand

Between 1917 and 1921, a number of cases were reported by several French neurologists — Marie et al.,[35] Roussey and Branche,[19] and Jumentié[19] — in which was described a "false ulnar claw hand" due to a "dissociated" lesion of the radial nerve. At first glance the resting attitude of the depicted hand resembled an ulnar claw because of the flexion attitude of the ring and little fingers at the metacarpophalangeal and interphalangeal joints. However, further inspection revealed that a true clawed digit with the usual hyperextension of the metacarpophalangeal joint was not present. This was confirmed when it was noted that all the ulnar-innervated intrinsic muscles were functioning. It was solely the extrinsic digital extensors to the ring and little fingers innervated by the posterior interosseous nerve that were partially paralyzed. A similar attitude of the hand can be seen in laceration of the long extensors of the third, fourth and fifth fingers (Fig. 33C) or in ruptures, as in rheumatoid arthritis (the Vaughan-Jackson syndrome) (Fig. 32).

Variations of Guyon's Tunnel

Several muscular variations have been noted at the level of Guyon's tunnel. These variations have clinical significance both as causative factors in low ulnar neuritic symptomatology and in the understanding of an anomalous operative field.

Variations of Guyon's tunnel are frequently associated with variations of the palmaris longus. When there is complete reversal of the usual muscle relationship of the palmaris longus (Fig. 128A),[47] the palmaris tendon arises proximally from the medial epicondyle, and its muscular belly attaches to the flexor retinaculum at the wrist. There is frequently an accessory slip, 1 cm. in thickness, which inserts into the pisiform. An arch (Fig. 128B) is thus created in the palmaris longus through which the ulnar nerve and artery penetrate into the wrist, running their normal course deep to the palmaris brevis. The ulnar nerve is in its usual location, medial to the ulnar artery.

Another muscular variation, noted by Schjelderup,[45] is of an anoma-

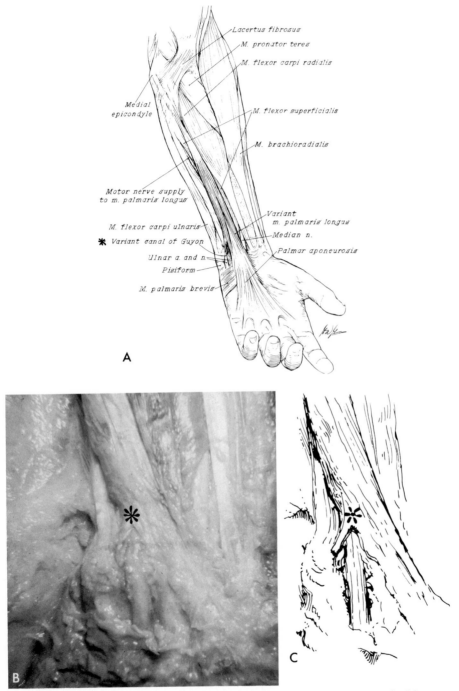

Figure 128.   *A*, Line drawing of a left anatomical specimen that presented with a completely reversed palmaris longus. There was a variation in the region of the canal of Guyon (*). *B*, The variant canal of Guyon (*) is demonstrated. A muscular slip of the reversed palmaris longus arose from the region of the pisiform. This muscular slip reinforced the roof of the tunnel. The ulnar nerve and artery are seen to pass posterior to this accessory muscular slip. *C*, Sketch of the variant Guyon canal (*) region.

lous muscle, 4 mm. wide, running in Guyon's tunnel and crossing the nerve before it divides. Turner and Caird[57] have described an anomalous muscle crossing Guyon's tunnel which passed between the motor and sensory branches. It arose from the pisiform and inserted into the transverse carpal ligament.

In a third type, Thomas[55] reported an anomalous accessory palmaris muscle, 1 cm. wide, which arose from the palmaris longus tendon and inserted in the region of the hypothenar muscles and, in part, the pisiform. This anomalous muscle passed through Guyon's tunnel. It gave clinical symptoms of easy fatigability of the hand. Dr. Kaplan[22] had dissected one anatomical specimen in which this anomalous muscle arose from the tendon of the flexor carpi ulnaris and inserted into the volar carpal ligament. It formed a thickened roof of Guyon's tunnel.

King and O'Rahilly[23] have reported a duplication of the palmaris longus with either a separate muscular slip (accessory palmaris) or tendon going from the duplicated palmaris and the abductor digiti quinti or the flexor digiti quinti. The accessory muscle passed anterior to the ulnar nerve and artery to reinforce the roof of Guyon's tunnel. On occasion the tendinous slip can interpose between the ulnar artery and nerve, with the artery crossing it superficially. Further association of anomalous palmaris longus and variations in the region of Guyon's tunnel have been reported by Wood.[62] A high origin of the flexor digiti quinti from a palmaris longus having a double origin was noted. Jeffery[18] has documented an accessory abductor digiti quinti as a cause of isolated paralysis of the intrinsics without sensory involvement. The variant muscle arose from the fascia of the lower forearm. The patient's symptoms were improved following excision of the hypertrophied muscle mass. Swanson[54] identified an accessory flexor digiti quinti arising from the forearm fascia, inserting into the flexor digitorum brevis, and causing symptoms of ulnar nerve compression.

Lipscomb[32] reported a case of duplication of the hypothenar muscles which simulated a tumor of the hand. The origin of the anomalous muscle was the pisiform and the hook of the hamate. The palmaris brevis was six times normal size. Proximally, these anomalous muscles formed part of the roof of Guyon's tunnel.

Hayes, Mulholland and O'Connor[15] have described a ligamentous band which runs from the pisiform to the hook of the hamate anterior to the deep branch of the ulnar nerve. The flexor and abductor digiti minimi muscles arise in part from this structure (Fig. 129). The abductor digiti minimi may be functioning if its motor branch arises from the ulnar nerve proximal to this ligamentous band in a paralysis of the motor branch of the ulnar nerve in this region. Additional pathological factors such as ganglia (Fig. 130 B–D), rheumatoid synovitis (Fig. 131), localized

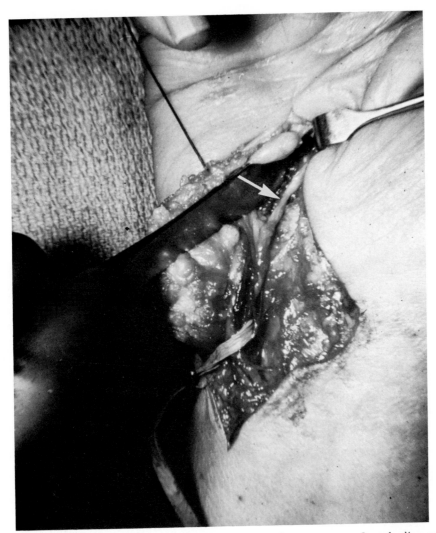

Figure 129.   Compression of the deep branch of the ulnar nerve was found adjacent to the hook of the hamate. There was narrowing of the nerve. No local pathology other than the ligamentous band described by Hayes et al. was found. Function in the intrinsic muscles returned 6 months after the neurolysis.

osteoarthritis, Dupuytren's contracture,[24] aneurysm, arteritis, fracture of the hamate, anomalous muscles,[59] anomalous deep branch of the ulnar nerve,[26, 27] and trauma can be present in this type of entrapment. In addition to classic occupation-induced traumatic neuritis, ulnar neuropathy caused by prolonged bicycling has recently been reported.[7] Hyper-

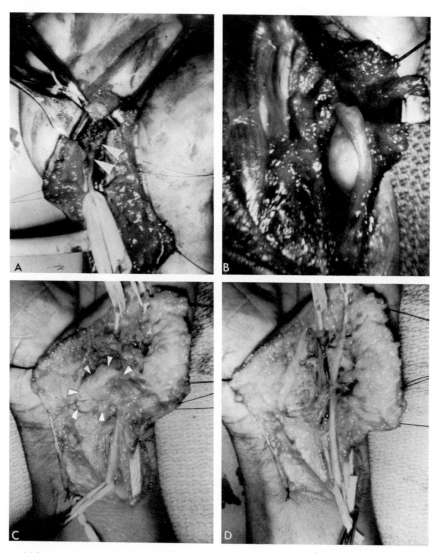

Figure 130.   *A*, Right hand. The ulnar nerve is in the Penrose drain; a neuroma and an adjacent glioma were noted in the deep branch of the ulnar nerve. Sensation was intact in the ring and little fingers. *B*, A ganglion displacing the ulnar nerve was found in the canal of Guyon of this left hand, causing low ulnar motor and sensory disturbances in the hand. The ganglion arose from the adjacent intercarpal joint. *C*, Left hand. A ganglion arose from the palmar aponeurosis which produced only sensory dysfunction in the ring and little fingers. *D*, The compression of the sensory branches occurred distal to the deep motor ulnar branch.

trophied flexor carpi ulnaris muscle in close proximity to Guyon's tunnel can also cause ulnar neuropathy.[14]

If a more proximal lesion is present in Guyon's tunnel, the clinical picture is that of low ulnar nerve lesion with loss of sensation in the volar aspect of the ulnar 1½ digits and intrinsic muscle loss (including the abductor digiti quinti) but with normal sensation in the region supplied by the ulnar dorsal cutaneous nerve. Kopell and Thompson,[25] Nicolle and Woolhouse,[38] and Torok and Giora[56] have reported similar anatomical findings.

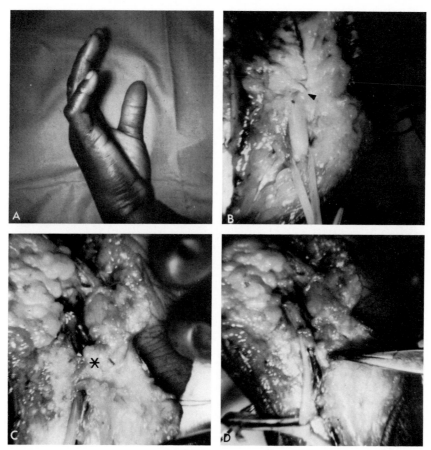

Figure 131. Low ulnar nerve paralysis (sensory and motor) associated with median nerve involvement in a rheumatoid right hand. *A*, Note the fullness of the palm in the hypothenar and carpal tunnel region. The hand has the attitude of an ulnar nerve paralysis. *B*, The median nerve is shown constricted proximal to the carpal tunnel (arrow). *C*, The asterisk denotes the level of the canal of Guyon. The ulnar nerve and its accompanying blood vessels pass through this canal. *D*, The hemostat denotes the thickened roof of the tunnel which has been released.

OPERATIVE APPROACH TO THE ULNAR NERVE IN THE FOREARM

The ulnar nerve is exposed with relative ease throughout its course. It runs in a straight line from the posterior aspect of the medical epicondyle to the pisiform (Fig. 132). It can be identified throughout its course when full exposure is required. Just proximal to the medial epi-

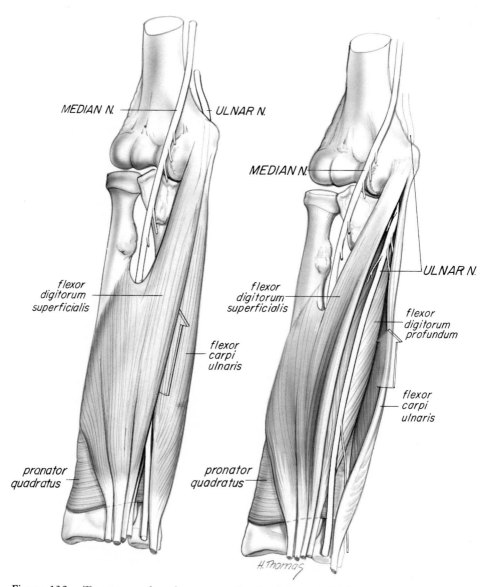

Figure 132. To expose the ulnar nerve in the forearm the internervous plane that needs to be developed is between the flexor carpi ulnaris and the flexor digitorum superficialis.

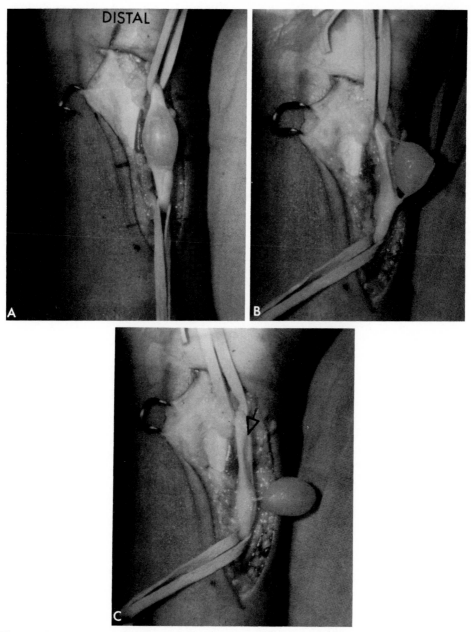

Figure 133. *A*, A neurilemoma of the ulnar nerve was accurately exposed in the lower fourth of this left forearm. *B*, The solitary funiculus involved in the pathological process is visualized. *C*, The groove (arrow) caused by the tumor in the ulnar nerve is noted. Full sensory and motor function in the hand was observed postoperatively.

condyle, and posterior to the distal humerus, there is one small articular branch (which can be sacrificed if necessary). The branches to the flexor carpi ulnaris and the flexor digitorum profundus must be preserved; they are identified after the aponeurosis over the cubital tunnel is incised. The two or three branches to the flexor carpi ulnaris and the usual single branch of the flexor profundus of the fourth and fifth fingers are easily identified. The origin of the flexor carpi ulnaris is split at its proximal end just distal to the elbow. Near the wrist the fascia over the flexor carpi ulnaris is incised proximal to the pisiform.

After the tendon is retracted ulnarly, the ulnar nerve and artery are identified in the same plane deep to the tendon. The nerve is located medial to the artery with its venae comitantes. The nerve can be traced proximally. The dorsal cutaneous nerve is identified as it arises from the ulnar side of the nerve approximately 6 to 8 cm. proximal to the ulnar styloid; it comes up under the medial border of the flexor carpi ulnaris tendon about 1 cm. proximal to the ulnar styloid. Occasionally, as the ulnar nerve is traced more proximally, a branch to the flexor carpi ulnaris may be found in the midforearm.

Ulnar nerve pathology can be accurately evaluated and the patient can be given optimal care when this anatomical approach to the nerve is utilized (Fig. 133).

BIBLIOGRAPHY

1. Apfelberg, D.B., and Larson, S.J.: Dynamic Anatomy of the Ulnar Nerve at the Elbow. Plast. Reconstr. Surg., 51:76–81, 1973.
2. Brooks, D.M.: Nerve Compression by Simple Ganglia. J. Bone Joint Surg., 34B:391–400, 1952.
3. Cannieu, J.M.A.: Recherches sur une Anastomose Entre la Branche Profunde du Cubitale et le Médian. Bull. Soc. d'Anat. Physiol. Bordeaux, 18:339–340, 1897.
4. Childress, H.M.: Recurrent Ulnar-Nerve Dislocation at the Elbow. Clin. Orthop., 108:168–173, 1975.
5. Denman, E.E.: An Unusual Branch of the Ulnar Nerve in the Hand. Hand, 9:92–93, 1977.
6. Dupont, C., Cloutier, G.E., Prevost, Y., and Dion, M.A.: Ulnar-Tunnel Syndrome at the Wrist. J. Bone Joint Surg., 47A:757–761, 1965.
7. Eckman, P.B., Perlstein, G., and Altrocchi, P.H.: Ulnar Neuropathy in Bicycle Riders. Arch. Neurol., 32:130–131, 1975.
8. Ehrlich, G.E.: Antecubital Cysts in Rheumatoid Arthritis—A Corollary to Popliteal (Baker's) Cysts. J. Bone Joint Surg., 54A:165–169, 1972.
9. Feindel, W., and Stratford, J.: The Role of the Cubital Tunnel in Tardy Ulnar Palsy. Can. J. Surg., 1:296, 1958.
10. Fragiadakis, E.G., and Lamb, D.W.: An Unusual Cause of Ulnar Nerve Compression. Hand, 2:14–15, 1970.
11. Freundlich, B.D., and Spinner, M.: Nerve Compression Syndrome in Derangements of the Proximal and Distal Radioulnar Joints. Bull. Hosp. Joint Dis., 19:38–47, 1968.
12. Grigoresco, M., and Iordanesco, C.: Un Case Rare de Paralysie Partielle du Nerf Radial. Rev. Neurol., 2:102–104, 1931.
13. Guyon, F.: Note sur une Disposition Anatomique Propre à la Face Antérieure de la Région du Poignet et non Encores Décrite par le Docteur. Bull. Soc. Anat. Paris, 2nd series. 6:184–186, 1861.
14. Harrelson, J.M., and Newman, M.: Hypertrophy of the Flexor Carpi Ulnaris as a Cause of Ulnar-Nerve Compression in the Distal Part of the Forearm. Case Report. J. Bone Joint Surg., 57A:554–555, 1975.

15. Hayes, J.R., Mulholland, R.C., and O'Connor, B.T.: Compression of the Deep Palmar Branch of the Ulnar Nerve. J. Bone Joint Surg., *51B:*469–472, 1969.
16. Henle, J.: Handbuch der Systematichen Anatomie des Menschen. Braunschweig, Vieweg, 1868.
17. Howard, F.M.: Ulnar-Nerve Palsy in Wrist Fractures. J. Bone Joint Surg., *43A:*1197–1201, 1961.
18. Jeffery, A.K.: Compression of the Deep Palmar Branch of the Ulnar Nerve by an Anomalous Muscle. J. Bone Joint Surg., *53B:*718–723, 1971.
19. Jumentié, M.J.: Fausse Griffe Cubitale par Lésion Dissociée du Nerf Radial. Rev. Neurol., *37:*755–758, 1921.
20. Kane, E., Kaplan, E.B., and Spinner, M.: Observations of the Course of the Ulnar Nerve in the Arm. Ann. Chir., *27:*487–496, 1973
21. Kaplan, E.B.: Variation of the Ulnar Nerve at the Wrist. Bull. Hosp. Joint Dis., *24:*85–88, 1963
22. Kaplan, E.B.: Personal Communcation, 1968.
23. King, T.S., and O'Rahilly, R.: M. Palmaris Accessorius and Duplication of M. Palmaris Longus. Acta Anat., *10:*327–331, 1950.
24. Kleinert, H.E., and Hayes, J.R.: The Ulnar Tunnel Syndrome. Plast. Reconstr. Surg., *47:*21–24, 1971.
25. Kopell, H.P., and Thompson, W.A.: Peripheral Entrapment Neuropathies. Baltimore, Williams & Wilkins, 1963.
26. Lanz, U.: Lahmung des Tiefen Hohlhandastes des Nervus Ulnaris, bedingt durch eine Anatomische Variante. Handchirurigie, *6:*83–86, 1974.
27. Lassa, R., and Shrewsbury, M.M.: A Variation in the Path of the Deep Motor Branch of the Ulnar Nerve at the Wrist. J. Bone Joint Surg., *57A:* 990–991, 1975.
28. Learmonth, J.R.: A Variation in the Distribution of the Radial Branch of the Musculospiral Nerve. J. Anat., *53:*371–372, 1919.
29. Learmonth, J.R.: Technique for Transplanting the Ulnar Nerve. Surg. Gynecol. Obstet., *75:* 792–793, 1942.
30. LeDouble, A.F.: Traité des Variations du Système Musculaire de l'Homme. Paris, Schleicher, 1897.
31. Leffert, R.D., and Dorfman, H.D.: Antecubital Cyst in Rheumatoid Arthritis. Surgical Findings. J. Bone Joint Surg., *54A:*1555–1557, 1972.
32. Lipscomb, P.R.: Duplication of Hypothenar Muscles Simulating Soft-tissue Tumor of the Hand. J. Bone Joint Surg., *42A:*1058–1061, 1960.
33. Liveson, J.A., Ranschoff, J., and Goodgold, J.: Electromyographic Studies in a Case of Foramen Magnum Meningioma. J. Neurol. Neurosurg. Psychiat. *36:*561–564, 1973.
34. Mannerfelt, L.: Studies on the Hand in Ulnar Nerve Paralysis. A Clinical-Experimental Investigation in Normal and Anomalous Innervation, Acta Orthop. Scand. Suppl., 87, 1966.
35. Marie, P., Meige, H., and Patrikios: Paralysie Radiale Dissociée Simulant une Griffe Cubitale. Rev. Neurol., *24:*123–124, 1917.
36. McFarlane, R.M., Mayer, J.R., and Hugill, J.V.: Further Observations on the Anatomy of the Ulnar Nerve at the Wrist. Hand, *8:*115–117, 1976.
37. Neblett, C., and Ehni, G.: Medial Epicondylectomy for Ulnar Palsy. J. Neurosurg., *32:*55–62, 1970.
38. Nicolle, F.V., and Woolhouse, F.M.: Nerve Compression Syndromes of the Upper Limb. J. Trauma, *5:*313–318, 1965.
39. Osborne, G.: The Surgical Treatment of Tardy Ulnar Neuritis. J. Bone Joint Surg., *39B:*782, 1957.
40. Osborne, G.: Compression Neuritis of the Ulnar Nerve at the Elbow. Hand, *2:*10–13, 1970.
41. Poirier, P., and Charpy, A.: Traité d'Anatomie Humaine. Vol. 3, Paris, Masson, 1901.
42. Riche, P.: Le Nerf Cubital et les Muscles de l'Eminence Thenar. Bull. Mem. Soc. Anat. Paris, *5:*251–252, 1897.
43. Rolfsen, L.: Snapping Triceps Tendon with Ulnar Neuritis. Acta Orthop. Scand., *41:*74–76, 1970.
44. Roussy, G., and Branche, J.: Deux Cas de Paralysies Dissociées de la Branche Postérieure du Radial, à Type de Pseudo-Griffe Cubitale. Rev. Neurol., *24:*312–314, 1917.
45. Schjelderap, H.: Aberrant Muscle in the Hand Causing Ulnar Nerve Compression. J. Bone Joint Surg., *46B:*361, 1964.
46. Shea, J.D., and McClain, E.J.: Ulnar Nerve Compression Syndromes at and below the Wrist. J. Bone Joint Surg., *51A:*1095–1103, 1969.
47. Spinner, M., and Freundlich, B.D.: An Important Variation of the Palmaris Longus. Bull. Hosp. Joint Dis., *28:*126–130, 1967.
48. Spinner, M., and Kaplan, E.B.: The Relationship of the Ulnar Nerve to the Medial Intermuscular Septum in the Arm and Its Clinical Significance. Hand, *8:*239–242, 1976.

49. Struthers, J.: On a Peculiarity of the Humerus and Humeral Artery. Monthly J. Med. Sci., *8*:264–267, 1848.
50. Struthers, J.: On Some Points in the Abnormal Anatomy of the Arm. Br. Foreign Medico-Chirurgical Review, *14*:170–179, 1854.
51. Struthers, J.: Anatomical and Physiological Observations. Part I, Edinburgh, Sutherland and Knox, 1854.
52. Sunderland, S.: The Innervation of the Flexor Digitorum Profundus and Lumbrical Muscles. Anat. Rec., *93*:317–321, 1945.
53. Sunderland, S.: Nerves and Nerve Injuries. Baltimore, Williams & Wilkins Co., 1968, p. 749.
54. Swanson, A.B., Biddulph, S.L., Baughman, F.A., and De Groot, G.: Ulnar Nerve Compression due to an Anomalous Muscle in the Canal of Guyon. Clin. Orthop., *83*:64–69, 1972.
55. Thomas, C.G.: Clinical Manifestations of an Accessory Palmaris Muscle. J. Bone Joint Surg., *40A*:929–930, 1958.
56. Torok, G., and Giora, A.: Ulnar Nerve Lesion in the Palm. Entrapment Neuropathy of the Deep Branch of the Ulnar Nerve. Israel Med. J., *23*:121–128, 1964.
57. Turner, M.S., and Caird, D.M.: Anomalous Muscles and Ulnar Nerve Compression at the Wrist. Hand, *9*:140–142, 1977.
58. Turner, W.: Further Examples of Variations in the Arrangement of the Nerves of the Human Body. J. Anat. Physiol., *8*:299, 1874.
59. Uriburu, I.J.F., Morchio, F.J., and Marin, J.C.: Compression Syndrome of the Deep Branch of the Ulnar Nerve. (Piso-Hamate Hiatus Syndrome). J. Bone Joint Surg., *58A*:145–147, 1976.
60. Vanderpool, D.W., Chalmers, J., Lamb, D.W., and Whiston, T.B.: Peripheral Compression Lesions of the Ulnar Nerve. J. Bone Joint Surg., *50B*: 792–803, 1968.
61. Wadsworth, T.G.: The External Compression Syndrome of the Ulnar Nerve at the Cubital Tunnel. Clin. Orthop., *124*:189–204, 1977.
62. Wood, J.: On Some Varieties in Human Myologies. Proc. Roy. Soc. Lond., *13*:299–303, 1864.

Section XI

SUMMARY

SUMMARY

This text has presented the results of a 20-year study made by the author of injuries to major branches of the peripheral nerves in the forearm. It correlates clinical experience with anatomical dissections in an effort to develop a better understanding of the various patterns of dysfunction that are observed when these branches are damaged.

A presentation of the resting and pinch attitudes of the hand has been made, and the diagnosis of specific injury to the major branches has been confirmed by evaluation of the status of other muscles innervated by these nerves. The appearance of the injured hands presents patterns of dysfunction which are quite different from those usually seen in complete median, radial, or ulnar nerve lesions. Recognition of these attitudes of the hand makes it possible to perform prompt primary repair of lacerated branches of major nerves. In addition, early release of an entrapped major branch should be completed before the muscles involved have gone on to irreversible atrophy or the internal neural fibrosis has extended to produce a neuroma-in-continuity. With timely recognition of these pathological attitudes, the need for prompt surgical intervention becomes evident.

My personal experience has led me to believe that these branches can best be repaired in the primary period. Otherwise, the following problems arise during secondary surgical repair: scarring of the wound, inability to make up nerve gaps, and especially, concern about adding further loss of function during the secondary dissection with excision of neuromata. Difficult surgical decisions as regards the extent of neuroma in partially injured nerves can be avoided by adopting the policy of primary repair where feasible.

Primary nerve suture can be expected to restore satisfactory function of the involved muscles. One can conclude that in managing these nerve lesions of the forearm it is better to restore the normal function to muscles which have been denervated than to perform primary tendon transfers. The best functional results can be anticipated by restoring the normal neuromuscular unit.

In summary, then, it has been my object to present the signs and concepts of management of lesions of major branches of the peripheral nerves of the forearm.

INDEX

Note: In this index, page numbers in *italic* type refer to illustrations; page numbers followed by (t) refer to tables.